RCGP AKT: Research, Epidemiology and Statistics

DR JULIAN HICK

General Practitioner
Chesterfield

and

DR RALPH EMMERSON

Programme Director
Chesterfield GP Training Programme
General Practitioner, Matlock

Foreword by
PROFESSOR MIKE PRINGLE

President
Royal College of General Practitioners

Radcliffe Publishing
London • New York

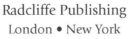

Radcliffe Publishing Ltd
St Mark's House
Shepherdess Walk
London N1 7BQ
United Kingdom

www.radcliffehealth.com

British Library Cataloguing in Publication Data

A catalogue record for this book is available from the British Library.

ISBN-13: 978 190936 811 8

The paper used for the text pages of this book is FSC® certified. FSC (The Forest Stewardship Council®) is an international network to promote responsible management of the world's forests.

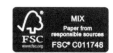

Typeset by Darkriver Design, Auckland, New Zealand
Manufacturing managed by 21six

Contents

Chapter 8: Conclusions   132

Chapter 9: Practice questions   140

Foreword by Professor Mike Pringle

To be a generalist is to accept a profound challenge. Our patients look to us to be clinically expert in everything and anything; to treat them in the round as people with specific needs and expectations; to know when to ask for help and advice; to be their confidential adviser; and to behave ethically at all times.

The more a doctor specialises, the more they know about a narrow field. As general practitioners we need to know enough about every area of medicine and much of anthropology, psychology and the other social sciences. To deliver safe care we must be good diagnosticians and careful prescribers, while tolerating a level of uncertainty. And to continually improve we need to reflect on our care, learning as we go and continually striving to maintain our standards.

This is no small ask!

Although we work in teams, our consultations are often one-to-one, private interactions that need to be conducted with humanity and skill. This makes us vulnerable to hubris and short cuts; to falling into bad habits and even burnout. A good new doctor needs to adopt techniques to guard against these risks.

One way to ensure that we embark on our general practice careers with the right attributes is through vocational training and the MRCGP examination. It is only a start, a launch pad, but it is an essential demonstration that we have the knowledge, clinical and social skills, and attitudes, suitable for a career in primary care.

The MRCGP has been meticulously designed to ensure that candidates are objectively assessed in these attributes for general practice. A key component of the MRCGP is the Applied Knowledge Test (AKT) that is the focus of this book.

Passing the AKT is, of course, part of the rite of passage into general practice, but it should be seen more as a way for a doctor to demonstrate that they have acquired the knowledge, and other skills, to be a safe and effective general practitioner.

Throughout your career, you will be reading research papers and applying new evidence to your practice. You will be puzzling over the ethics of sharing clinical information with managers and researchers. You will be looking at your clinical practice to see how it can be improved. For these tasks you need appropriate knowledge, the skills to apply it and the will to do so.

This book, written with verve and clarity, is therefore both a primer for the AKT and a guide to good practice. It will travel with you through your first decades in general practice as an aide-mémoire and a source of wisdom. It contains truths that will be your talismans and guides. I hope you enjoy it as much as I have.

Professor Mike Pringle
President
Royal College of General Practitioners
June 2014

About the authors

Dr Julian Hick

Julian came to medicine after spending several years working as an academic in the social sciences and humanities. He taught on several postgraduate and undergraduate courses but spent most time teaching research methods. During this time he also undertook research using both qualitative and quantitative methods, including research into gender, equality and socio-economic deprivation. He is now a general practitioner living and working in Derbyshire after completing the MRCGP in 2012. Additionally, he works in the Academic Unit of Primary Medical Care at the University of Sheffield. His academic interests include inequalities in health and healthcare, translating research into practice and, of course, teaching evidence-based medicine and statistics.

Dr Ralph Emmerson

Ralph is a Programme Director for the Chesterfield GP Training Programme and a full-time practising GP in Matlock, Derbyshire. He has held many educator roles over the years, from teaching undergraduates to experienced GPs. It was whilst Julian Hick was a trainee on the Chesterfield Training Programme, that a need for a better AKT statistics book was identified. Their collaboration has resulted in this book.

Acknowledgements

We are very grateful for helpful comments and suggestions from Chris Knight and Sarah Emmerson, which have undoubtedly improved this book. We are also grateful for the good-natured and unflagging support we have received during the writing of this manuscript from Jo, Sophie and Alex.

Not forgetting, too, the encouragement and interest of Ben and Ollie from their distant medical schools.

Thanks to Dr Chris Cates for permission to use the Cates plot, created via the free software Visual Rx available online at www.nntonline.net, shown in Chapter 7. Thanks also to Dr Petra Boynton for permission to use the table on improving response time for questionnaires in Chapter 4.

JH acknowledges the support and suggestions he has received from his colleagues at the Academic Unit of Primary Medical Care at the University of Sheffield.

While others have helped and made suggestions, any errors remain ours alone.

List of abbreviations

ACE-I	ACE inhibitor
AKT	Applied Knowledge Test
AR	absolute risk
ARI	absolute risk increase
ARR	absolute risk reduction
BNF	*British National Formulary*
CER	control event rate
CKD	chronic kidney disease
COC	combined oral contraceptive
DALY	disability-adjusted life year
DENs	doctor's educational needs
DVT	deep vein thrombosis
EER	experimental event rate
FN	false negative
FP	false positive
GI	gastrointestinal
GP	general practitioner
HR	hazard ratio
LR	likelihood ratio
MCQ	multiple-choice question
MHRA	Medicines and Healthcare Products Regulatory Agency
MMR	measles, mumps and rubella vaccination
MRCGP	Membership of the Royal College of General Practitioners
NHS	National Health Service
NICE	National Institute for Health and Care Excellence
NIHR	National Institute for Health Research
NNH	number needed to harm
NNT	number needed to treat
NPV	negative predictive value
NSAID	non-steroidal anti-inflammatory drug
OR	odds ratio

PPV	positive predictive value
PSA	prostate-specific antigen
PUN	patient's unmet need
QALY	quality-adjusted life year
RCGP	Royal College of General Practitioners
RCT	randomised controlled trial
RR	relative risk
RRI	relative risk increase
RRR	relative risk reduction
SEM	standard error of the mean
TN	true negative
TP	true positive

Introduction

EVIDENCE-BASED MEDICINE AND EVIDENCE-BASED PRACTICE

Doctors have a lot of responsibilities to their patients: a responsibility to make sure that they treat each patient with appropriate care and attention; a responsibility to make sure that they apply the best knowledge to their clinical practice; a responsibility to make sure that they are competent in their actions; a responsibility to avoid conflicts of interest that could adversely affect their patients. With this background it can be seen that using the best available evidence of what works is vital to good medical care.

Undergraduate medical courses normally include some lectures, workshops and discussions of evidence-based medicine. Moving from this knowledge acquisition to being a practitioner of evidence-based medicine can be tough. During those years of trying to assimilate a huge amount of information on basic sciences and clinical practice, critical appraisal and evidence-based medicine may take a back seat. It is often easier to learn from your senior colleagues, lecturers and peers than it is to evaluate the evidence yourself. The assumption is that many of these people know more than you and have greater experience. However, if you can maintain your critical appraisal skills and evidence-based practice it is likely that the care you give your patients will be improved.

Evidence-based medicine, as a movement or paradigm, has been around for some decades now, but initially it didn't have a big impact on the way doctors and other healthcare professionals practised. The origins of evidence-based practice as we understand it today can be traced back to pioneers such as Archie Cochrane and his realisation that clinicians needed much better information about what worked and what did not when treating their patients.[*]

It was in 1991 that the term 'evidence-based medicine' was probably first used, when Gordon Guyatt at McMaster University published an editorial in

---

[*] See Cochrane A, *Effectiveness and Efficiency: random reflections on health services.* London: Nuffield Provincial Hospitals Trust; 1972.

the *ACP Journal Club* titled 'Evidence-Based Medicine'.[*] He had earlier coined the term 'scientific medicine', but that had caused a furore and he had to change the term. His idea was that critical appraisal techniques should be used to improve the teaching of medical students and therefore also clinical care. Critical appraisal techniques were discussed in a series of articles in the *Canadian Medical Association Journal* in 1981, written by staff from McMaster University who had been teaching students based on patient problems, epidemiology and statistics. These were the building blocks on which Guyatt created evidence-based medicine teaching programmes at McMaster University in the 1990s.

Evidence-based medicine was formed against the backdrop of clinicians largely following the teaching of their seniors and respected experts or authorities, rather than any certain evidence. The costs of medical treatments were also increasing, as they continue to do, and using limited resources effectively was becoming more important. The pioneers of evidence-based medicine wanted to make sure that clinicians had access to good-quality evidence that could inform their clinical practice. Answering basic questions such as whether a treatment was more likely to harm or to help patients was seen to be necessary to improve clinical treatment and the cost-effectiveness of treatment.

When medicine is based on expert opinion it is very hard for junior clinicians to challenge their seniors. Where there is no evidence for treatments it falls to 'experts' to make decisions around which treatments to offer to patients. Evidence-based medicine aimed to turn this around so that decisions were based on evidence and therefore anyone could challenge accepted practice if he or she had good supporting evidence.

However, having good-quality evidence is only one part of evidence-based practice. It is also important that the preferences and needs of individual patients are taken into account when weighing up the evidence and deciding what treatment to undertake. This is why the term 'evidence-based practice' has become more commonplace, reflecting the fact that medicine is practised in alliance with patients and should not be something that is imposed on patients. As general practitioners (GPs) it is fundamental that we work in partnership with our patients in order to gain the most appropriate outcomes for them. We need to know the advantages and disadvantages of the treatments we offer to our patients so that we can share decision-making with them. This is, of course, in addition to our clinical experiences – we have to engage our clinical acumen as well as being aware of the best evidence.

Evidence-based medicine is not without its critics, and there are problems in translating critical appraisal to clinical practice. Some of these criticisms are considered in Chapter 8. In brief, the limits of evidence-based medicine are

---

[*] Guyatt GH. Evidence-based medicine. *ACP J Club*. 1991; 114: A–16.

felt where it is not possible to have good-quality evidence for particular patient groups, such as elderly people with several co-morbidities and who are already on a raft of medications. There is a paucity of research based on these patients due to the limitations of research methods such as randomised controlled trials and the difficulties in translating their outcomes to the individual patient in front of us. It takes a considerable amount of time (and money) to conduct a good randomised controlled trial and therefore the results may not be known for many months, or even years. Of even more importance is that the results of good trials are often not applied in clinical settings for many years. We still have some way to go before evidence-based medicine or evidence-based practice is able to deliver all the possible benefits that it could do.

Evidence-based medicine provides a firm foundation for our clinical practice and we need to engage with evidence in order to keep our practice up to date, safe and effective. It is to be hoped this book can help you to engage effectively with your patients based on evidence of what works.

ABOUT THIS BOOK

This book is primarily for GP trainees contemplating the Applied Knowledge Test (AKT). We hope that it will also be helpful to others who are interested in developing their knowledge and practice of evidence-based medicine. It is also about how to apply research findings to general practice. Everything in the book is directly related to the Royal College of General Practitioners (RCGP) curriculum. The curriculum is based on all the knowledge that a competent GP could be expected to have in order to practise safely and effectively.

The main aim of this book remains to help GP trainees pass the AKT, but as such it has some limitations. It does not aim to be a comprehensive introduction to evidence-based medicine or a guide for researchers. At times we have deliberately skimmed the surface, knowing we are avoiding particular debates or controversies, in order to keep the focus on the level of understanding that a candidate for the AKT needs to have.

You need to pass the AKT. It is one of the hurdles you need to get over before becoming fully qualified as a GP. The exam covers clinical medicine, administrative issues and, the part this book is concerned with, critical appraisal and evidence-based practice. The 10% of marks that are in the critical appraisal and evidence-based practice section could be the difference between failing and passing. This book aims to help you understand critical appraisal and evidence-based practice. Having this understanding should help you pick up marks on the AKT – the answers to the critical appraisal and evidence-based medicine questions are often relatively easy to work out if you have the right knowledge. There are many questions for you to practise, so that you can be sure you have assimilated the appropriate knowledge. Preparing effectively for the AKT will increase your chances of passing. This book aims to cover the topics in the critical appraisal and evidence-based medicine section of the RCGP *The Applied Knowledge Test Content Guide*, which is available on the RCGP website (www. rcgp.org.uk) and is something that you should certainly read. This book is one part of your preparation process.

It is also our hope that this book will provide you with the tools for critical appraisal and evidence-based practice that will underpin your clinical practice after you have become a fully qualified GP. Evidence-based medicine is extremely important for making sure that our patients receive the best, most appropriate and least harmful treatments. Therefore, being able to understand and evaluate the medical literature is essential. This is normally taught at medical undergraduate level but it can be neglected once the pressures of learning clinical medicine and performing the daily tasks of a junior doctor become more important. We hope in this book that we show how critical appraisal and evidence-based medicine are essential for good medical practice throughout your career. We do recognise that there are limits to evidence-based medicine and these are discussed throughout the text (in particular, *see* Chapter 8).

Chapter 1 is a brief introduction to the AKT, including how to prepare for the AKT. Much of this chapter applies to the whole AKT, not just the 10% on critical appraisal and evidence-based medicine. Questions are found throughout the subsequent chapters, including the final chapter entirely consisting of practice questions. The book will make sense to read from start to finish and you can do the practice questions as you go; the answers to most of the questions in each chapter are to be found in the text of that chapter. Alternatively, you could focus on the questions in the final chapter and if struggling to answer them correctly you can then turn back to the appropriate section of the book to revise that topic.

We cover a bit of background in Chapter 2, an introduction to statistics – this chapter discusses probability and statistical significance in particular. Inferential and descriptive statistics are explained, along with the sometimes confusing ideas of the null hypothesis and p-values. There is also a brief discussion on the limits of statistics – some things cannot be understood adequately with statistical analysis, or with statistical analysis alone. We also need to be aware that data may not be as useful as they appear – we cover the ideas of reliability, validity and generalisability in this chapter.

Basic descriptive statistics, correlation, confidence intervals and graphical representations of data are discussed in Chapter 3. This chapter also introduces the idea that there are different types of numerical data, all which need to be understood in order to see which statistical tests can be used to analyse data appropriately.

Chapter 4 turns away from statistics and quantitative methods to discuss qualitative methods. These methods are very helpful in gaining a deeper understanding of individuals or groups of people in terms of their values and experiences. Often qualitative research is viewed as inferior to quantitative research; it actually aims to find out something different from, but often equally as important as, that which can be studied with quantitative methods. More powerfully qualitative and quantitative methods can be used together to gain deeper understanding of a research topic.

Chapters 5 and 6 look at quantitative research methods and epidemiology, respectively. These two chapters introduce a lot of formulas and show relatively simple applications of these formulas so that you can get used to applying them. Chapter 5 discusses common research methods and research outcomes, including the hierarchical pyramid of study designs. Chapter 6 covers some of the useful tests that are used in epidemiological studies and also discusses measures of mortality and economic analyses.

In Chapter 7 we turn to look at how to answer questions relevant to primary care and the practice of research in primary care. Research ethics are also considered in this chapter. In Chapter 8, the final text chapter, we have a brief recap of how to succeed in the AKT and then we take a slightly more critical look at evidence-based medicine and consider how it, and medicine more generally, may change in the future. Finally, as already mentioned, Chapter 9 consists entirely of practice questions.

PASSING THE APPLIED KNOWLEDGE TEST

Reading this book suggests that you want to pass the AKT and have therefore decided to improve your chances by preparing as best you can for the exam. As mentioned earlier, this book can only be one part of your work towards passing the AKT. Chapter 1 gives a lot of pointers to how to prepare for the AKT. We would argue that you should gain much of the knowledge you need to pass your membership examinations through your training rotations, but it is important to be focused on what you need to know to practise as an independent GP throughout all your training.

Starting thinking about what you need as a GP and staying focused on general practice will help make sure that your training rotations prepare you for life after membership examinations. Remember that the work you put in to passing your AKT will also be relevant for the Clinical Skills Assessment, where knowing the evidence will help in scoring marks in the management of your cases. We wish you luck, both in the AKT and in your future career as an independent, knowledgeable, caring and thoughtful GP. Now, let us turn to look in more detail at the AKT exam and how to prepare for it.

CHAPTER 1

The Applied Knowledge Test

The Applied Knowledge Test came into being in August 2007 as one of the three components of the Membership of the Royal College of General Practitioners (MRCGP) mandatory licensing examination. The other two components are the Clinical Skills Assessment and the Workplace Based Assessment. The AKT is a 200-item multiple-choice test that will take you 3 hours to complete, and here is the first statistic: that is *54 seconds* per question! That is the *mean* time you will need to spend on each question. This will increase to a mean of 57 seconds per question, when the AKT duration extends to three hours and ten minutes. Now we are on our way!

Of these 200 multiple-choice items, approximately 80% (160 items) are on clinical medicine; 10% (20 items) are on ethics, legal issues and organisational structure; and the final 10% (20 items) are on critical appraisal and evidence-based clinical practice. It is that final 10% we are interested in here, and we hope that reading this book will maximise your score in this section. Remember, every correct answer gives you 0.5%! Gaining the full 10% on these items will make a big difference to your score and could be the difference between passing and failing.

APPLIED KNOWLEDGE TEST QUESTION FORMATS

Why 200 *items* rather than 200 questions? Well, you may know that there are nine different formats of AKT questions. Let us have a look at the nine formats.

1. **Single best answer**. This is often a scenario-based question where there is only one correct answer. The others, the Royal College of General Practitioners tells us, may be plausible but are not the most likely. You must pick the *most likely* correct answer.
2. **Extended matching questions**. These questions have a list of possible

options. There will be two or more scenarios and you must choose the best option for each scenario. Each of the options may be used more than once or not at all.

3. **Table or algorithm**. There may be a table or algorithm with some empty spaces. You will be given some options and will need to choose the best option for each empty space. Options may be used more than once or not at all.

4. **Picture or video**. There will be a picture or video and then a question. From a list of options, you will need to pick the *most likely* option.

5. **'Drag and drop'**. A 'drag and drop' question may be similar to the table or algorithm but, instead of selecting an option, you will be able to use the computer mouse to drag one of the options and drop it into an empty space.

6. **Data interpretation**. These questions will require you to interpret data from a piece of research or an audit. You will be expected to use and apply common statistical terms. This means *you need to know the common formulas and how to use them*.

7. **Free text**. Here you will not be able to guess. The answer to a question will need to be typed into the space provided – the answer may be a word or a number. These answers are checked manually in case there has been any misspelling.

8. **Rank ordering**. These questions have a list of options that you need to put in the correct order. There will be only one order that gives the correct answer.

9. **'Hotspots'**. These, along with free text questions, were new to the AKT in 2010. Hotspot questions allow you to click on a graphic. This may be to indicate the site of a clinical sign, for example.

Therefore, there may be fewer than 200 questions, with more than one *item* (i.e. required answer) for some of the questions.

Information about the question formats can be found at the RCGP website (www.rcgp.org.uk). If you click on 'Exams' and then 'MRCGP exam' you should be able to see the link to the 'Applied Knowledge Test' web page, or you can search for AKT in the search box at the top of the page. *It is essential that you read through this web page well before you sit the AKT.* It will also tell you everything you need to know about applying to sit the AKT, what you need to learn and how you are notified of your result. You should read this entire page and open up and read all the links too. By working through this book, you will experience most of the different question formats, so you will become used to answering the different styles of questions.

THE IMPORTANCE OF STATISTICS!

We hope you will not mind if we digress for a moment to reinforce the importance of statistics. A computer marks your AKT result, with your success being determined by a number of statistics. To make sure each AKT is comparable with the next, a calculation is performed that requires the **mean** and **standard deviation** of each test. You do not need to know about the calculation but you do need to understand mean and standard deviation. To create a fair pass mark, each set of AKT results undergoes another calculation to set the pass mark. This calculation will use **p-values**. Again, you do not need to worry about the calculation, but can you define what a p-value is? Whether you pass or fail depends upon it! This is to ensure that any variation in the difficulty of the questions between exams is taken into account in the pass mark. Is that it? Well, no. The marks from your AKT then go through another calculation to check how **reliable** the results are. Yes, you guessed it! You need to know about reliability too. So your knowledge of statistics becomes data that undergo statistical analysis. That feels a bit strange, but essentially statistics determine whether you can become a GP or not. Statistics are very important to you, not to mention your patients.

APPLIED KNOWLEDGE TEST PASS RATES

You can find most of what we have just mentioned by looking at the AKT feedback on the RCGP website. The first AKT (AKT 1) took place in November 2007 and there is feedback available online from this and each subsequent sitting. From the January 2010 AKT (AKT 8), the standards used to set the pass mark were raised to reflect changes in the selection process of trainees. But do not worry; have a look at some statistics from the last 5 years, outlined in Figure 1.1.

Date	Number	Pass mark	Pass rate (the percentage who passed)	Mean score of trainees in the 20 critical appraisal and evidence-based clinical practice questions
April 2012	AKT 15	68.8%	67.6%	70.2%
October 2012	AKT 16	69.8%	71.6%	69.8%
January 2013	AKT 17	66%	68.7%	66.9%
May 2013	AKT 18	68%	71.4%	76%
October 2013	AKT 19	67%	76.1%	69.4%

FIGURE 1.1 Applied Knowledge Test pass mark and pass rate statistics

Now that does not look so bad. In fact, we also know that the cumulative pass rate after three attempts at the AKT is 98%. However, as you know, these reassuring statistics only come with hard work and you only get four attempts in total, so do not relax too much just yet. Just to show how things changed after January 2010, Figure 1.2 gives the statistics from an AKT prior to that date.

Date	Number	Pass mark	Pass rate (the percentage who passed)	Mean score of trainees in the 20 critical appraisal and evidence-based clinical practice questions
October 2009	AKT 7	67.8%	80.7%	72.9%

FIGURE 1.2 Statistics for the Applied Knowledge Test held in October 2009 (AKT 7)

Remember to look at the AKT feedback on the RCGP website that also includes areas where trainees performed poorly. You can then tailor your revision to these areas as well as your own learning needs. Interestingly the evidence-based medicine section has often been identified as an area where candidates perform badly.

REVISING FOR THE APPLIED KNOWLEDGE TEST

So what else can you do to revise for the AKT? Well, you have this book for the critical appraisal and evidence-based clinical practice section of the exam. General suggestions for your clinical practice, which will help you prepare for the AKT, include the following:
- maintain your medical knowledge from day one of your GP training
- keep a list of things to look up and do it
- learn from debriefs; quiz your trainer
- keep a logbook of patient's unmet needs (PUNs) and doctor's educational needs (DENs)
- identify your weak spots and improve them
- read through the GP curriculum
- know National Institute for Health and Care Excellence guidance, especially for common disorders
- read Scottish Intercollegiate Guidelines Network guidance, especially for common disorders
- keep referring back to the Cochrane Library for evidence
- read the RCGP's journal *InnovAiT* from day one
- read the *BMJ* and *British Journal of General Practice* clinical reviews from day one
- read the *Drug and Therapeutics Bulletin* as often as you can, and use it to look things up

- go on a general update course
- refer frequently to the *British National Formulary* (the BNF, www.bnf.org) and learn common side effects; read the first few 'Guidance on Prescribing' chapters
- understand the different consultation models
- know *Good Medical Practice*[*] and other important General Medical Council publications
- know about consent including General Medical Council guidance
- know about monitoring drugs such as disease-modifying anti-rheumatic drugs, amiodarone and lithium
- know the basics about benefits
- know the basics about sick certification
- know the Driver and Vehicle Licensing Agency's *At a Glance Guide to the Current Medical Standards of Fitness to Drive*[†]
- know about travel health and fitness to fly
- know about immunisation schedules and which are live vaccines
- know what the practice nurses do and how they follow the guidelines
- know about death certification and cremation forms
- know the basics of the Mental Health Act 1983
- know the basics of the Mental Capacity Act 2005.

Suggestions of specific things that you should do to prepare for the AKT include:
- read *all* the information on the RCGP AKT web page
- read through *The Applied Knowledge Test Content Guide*,[‡] available on the RCGP website
- working in groups can help share the workload, particularly when looking up guidelines
- work through online multiple-choice questions (MCQs) and possibly MCQ books; keep practising and make sure you learn from the questions you get wrong
- work through the RCGP essential knowledge challenges available online at http://elearning.rcgp.org.uk
- work through some modules from the e-GP website (run in partnership with the RCGP) at www.e-LfH.org.uk
- work through the Faculty of Sexual and Reproductive Healthcare

---

[*] General Medical Council. *Good Medical Practice*. London: GMC; 2013. Available at: www.gmc-uk.org/guidance/good_medical_practice.asp

[†] Drivers Medical Group. *At a Glance Guide to the Current Medical Standards of Fitness to Drive*. Swansea: DVLA; 2014. Available at: www.gov.uk/government/publications/at-a-glance

[‡] Royal College of General Practitioners. *The Applied Knowledge Test Content Guide*. London: RCGP; 2013. Available at: www.rcgp.org.uk/gp-training-and-exams/mrcgp-exam-overview/mrcgp-applied-knowledge-test-akt.aspx

e-learning modules to learn about sexual health www.e-lfh.org.uk/programmes/sexual-and-reproductive-healthcare/
- try to guess which algorithms may be used; think of chronic diseases, breast lumps, prostate cancer, menorrhagia
- read the *Oxford Handbook of General Practice** – especially the first 100 pages
- sit down with the practice manger and find out about health and safety, risk management, employment law
- know about the different GP contracts
- keep flash cards of important things or those things you forget easily.

There is a lot to do and the earlier you get started the better. Some of this you will do as part of your everyday work, but you will also have to focus specifically on the AKT to make sure you do not have any big gaps in your knowledge. The AKT is what it says on the tin. You need to have the knowledge but you also need to be able to apply it. The more work you do and the more you learn and apply your knowledge, the more likely you are to pass the AKT at your first attempt. Happily, this should also help you develop your clinical practice and set you up for a successful career in general practice.

PREPARATION FOR THE APPLIED KNOWLEDGE TEST

Before we move on to study statistics, critical appraisal and evidence-based medicine in more detail, here are some useful hints for when you are preparing for the exam.
- Make sure you read the information on the RCGP website so you know exactly what you need to take and what you need to do
- Work through the tutorial on the Pearson VUE website (www.pearsonvue.com) to get to know the computer screen layout
- Visit the Pearson VUE centre where you are going to take the AKT
- Do a test run from your home to the centre so you know the timing and the route
- If you get very nervous, talk to somebody (your GP?) about this
- Try to sleep well before the exam and relax

Finally, the following are some things to consider on the day of the exam and during the exam:
- make sure you arrive in good time
- make sure you do not drink too much caffeine

---

* Simon C, Everitt H, van Dorp F, Burkes M. *Oxford Handbook of General Practice*. 4th ed. Oxford: OUP; 2014.

- time management is absolutely crucial; keep a close eye on the clock showing the time remaining
- see if you can get the answer before you look at the options
- answer all the remaining questions; do not leave any unanswered; use an educated guess; the exam is not negatively marked
- review all the questions you did not answer first time, particularly answering those you feel you probably know the answer to.

One important point to make here is that *The Applied Knowledge Test Content Guide* does change with time. Do check the RCGP website to see if the guide has been updated since you started your revision. It is also worth knowing that there are a few areas from the research, statistics and epidemiology section of the guide that we could not include here. Examples of these are the main reasons for patients consulting in the UK and the health needs of special groups. This information should be gathered as you do your revision for the clinical component of the AKT.

So now we are ready to proceed. Enjoy this book and do not forget that what you are learning is not only important for your AKT but also important for your clinical practice as an evidence-based future GP.

CHAPTER 2

Basic statistics

INTRODUCTION TO STATISTICS

A patient comes in to see you and asks about the effectiveness of a contraceptive treatment that you suggest to her. Or more bluntly, 'Is this going to work? What is the risk of getting pregnant?' How do you answer this? When a patient comes in and asks, 'Should I have this PSA test?' what do you need to know in order to answer? In both of these scenarios, what you tell the patient can have a great impact on his or her decision. In order for your patient to make the best decision, he or she will need to know from you (1) what the most effective options are, (2) the risks and benefits for each option and (3) the chance of each risk and benefit occurring.

The very idea of 'statistics' can be instantly off-putting to many people. Statistics may be seen as a monolithic branch of mathematics filled with equations that may inform but only to those who understand complex equations. Statistics often seems to be taught in such a way that it does not seem related to the world around us but rather is mired in complicated techniques and produces outputs that are difficult (or impossible) to apply to an individual patient. The first bit of good news is that you do not need to be a mathematical genius to be able to use and interpret statistics. Second, you do not need to be able to understand or know complex equations. Third, statistics can be taught in a way that is interesting, relevant to our everyday work and helpful to both us and our patients.

Statistics give us a way of summarising the complex world around us. Statistics give us a way of comparing things that are similar in some way. We frequently use statistics – they inform a lot of our decisions at work and in our lives outside work. But how well do we use statistics? Do we use them with the subtlety of someone who truly understands them or do we use them uncritically and do we too easily accept what we are told? Understanding statistics and being able to evaluate evidence is a core skill that GPs need in order to provide the best quality care.

Now to the first practice questions in this book. The answers to these questions will be found in the text that follows. We start off with some definitions that you need to know and understand.

Q 2.1   If a study quotes a result with a 95% confidence interval, which one of the following statements is *true*?
a) There is a 95% chance of the true value lying outside these limits.
b) There is a 5% chance of the true value lying outside these limits.
c) There is a 2.5% chance of the true value lying outside these limits.
d) There is a minus 5% chance of the true value lying outside these limits.
e) There is a 5% chance that the study is flawed in its design.

Q 2.2   Which of the following definitions best applies to the term 'statistical significance'?
a) The result of a study is applicable to a selected population.
b) The result of a study is unlikely to have arisen by chance alone.
c) The result of a study is likely to be accurate.
d) The result of a study is not affected by chance.
e) The result of a study is within expected limits.

WHY UNDERSTANDING STATISTICS IS IMPORTANT

People widely view statistics with suspicion and distrust, but statistics themselves do not lie. 'Statistics' simply refers to the collection, analysis, interpretation and presentation of data. What they represent can be misinterpreted, inaccurately reported and misunderstood. Also statistics may not be measuring something in an accurate or appropriate way.

Understanding statistical techniques and being able to critique the presentation of research findings can help ensure that you are less likely to be misled. This is particularly important when you are using the results to treat your patients and can inform them of the options, risks and benefits.

There are many examples of statistical inferences being misused in medicine. A tragic and well-known example of this is the evidence presented in court by a respected paediatrician regarding the likelihood of a mother having two infants who unexpectedly die, without an appropriate explanation – so-called 'sudden infant death syndrome' (SIDS or cot death). This evidence was used to convict solicitor and mother Sally Clark of killing two of her children, a conviction that was later overturned largely due to more careful analysis of the statistical evidence.

The chance of one cot death was reported as 1 in 8543. The court was told that therefore the chance of two cot deaths in the same family was 1 in 73 million (8543 multiplied by 8543). This missed the point that after a family has been affected by one cot death the risk of a second cot death is much higher, at about 1 in 200.* Multiplying the risk of one cot death by itself would only be appropriate if both deaths were truly independent of each other.

The risk of a second cot death is actually much greater, because the family is still subject to the same risk factors that may have contributed to the first death. Therefore, the risk of a further cot death is not independent of the first. Eventually, after two appeals, Sally Clark was found not guilty. Tragically, she was found dead at her home 4 years after her release from prison. Careful application of statistics matters and in this case may have prevented an unnecessary death.

So statistics can be misused, but they are also vital for improving care and are the basis for evidence-based practice, both of which are compelling reasons to make sure statistics are better understood. Medical systems today collect massive quantities of statistics on how patients are treated, by whom and the outcomes of that treatment. These data are only useful if analysed and understood and appropriate action is then taken. This is why the AKT has a section on 'critical appraisal and evidence-based clinical practice' and why this book will provide you with the skills not only to help you to do well in your AKT but also to be a more effective and confident GP.

Q 2.3 Which of the following statements are *true* regarding descriptive statistics?
a) They are used to summarise the characteristics of study participants.
b) They give results from a sample group that are generalisable to the whole population.
c) They include methods such as the chi-squared test, regression and analysis of variance.
d) They include methods such as averages, measures of spread and deviation.
e) They are useful if you do not need to apply the results of your study to a larger population.

---

* See, among others, Watkins SJ. Conviction by mathematical error? Doctors and lawyers should get probability theory right. *BMJ.* 2000; **320**(7226): 2–3.

Q 2.4 Which of the following statements are *true* regarding inferential statistics?
a) They are used to summarise the characteristics of study participants.
b) They give results from a sample group that are generalisable to the whole population.
c) They include methods such as the chi-squared test, regression and analysis of variance.
d) They include methods such as averages, measures of spread and deviation.
e) They are useful if you wish to apply the results of your study to a larger population.

Q 2.5 Choose the best definition for 'null hypothesis' from the following options.
a) The wrong hypothesis
b) The hypothesis that the research will not produce a statistically significant result
c) The hypothesis that the results of a study are inaccurate
d) The hypothesis that there is no relationship between the study variables
e) The hypothesis that there is a relationship between the study variables

WHAT ARE STATISTICS?

Statistics are observations that are used to predict what processes have led to those observations. Probability is knowing how likely an event is, given knowledge about pre-existing conditions. For example, if we know how many people have a particular disease, then what is the chance that an individual chosen at random will have the disease? So probability is deductive whereas statistics use inductive processes to deal with uncertainty. Likelihood is a related concept: it is a measure of the extent to which a sample provides support for particular values of a population parameter.

Statistics can be broadly split into two types: descriptive statistics and inferential statistics. At the most fundamental level statistics are a numerical description of something quantifiable. These are descriptive statistics. Statistics can also be a statement of *probability: the chance of an event occurring given certain parameters*. These are inferential statistics. Both types of statistics can be very useful, but to infer something goes beyond simple description to look at how what is found in a study may apply beyond the sample of that study. It is this that makes inferential statistics so useful and interesting.

DESCRIPTIVE STATISTICS

The most commonly used descriptive statistic is probably the average. In everyday life we use averages to enable us to understand phenomena and to predict things. For example, knowing our average score on past papers of the AKT and comparing this with the average pass mark from previous papers is useful in guiding revision and knowing when we should sit the exam.

Descriptive statistics summarise data and enable quicker understanding of what the data represent. Describing data sets is important in allowing us to understand how representative the data set is of the population we are interested in. For example, the average age of study participants may be very different from the average age of patients we see and treat with the drug being studied. For this reason you should look at the descriptive statistics in a research paper (when they are provided) before the inferential statistical analysis.

Note that the use of the word 'population' does not necessarily mean the whole population of a country in this context. Instead, it refers to a specific group of individuals, or phenomena, that are of interest. Thus a population for a study of factors affecting male fertility may be males of reproductive age within a particular geographical area.

Descriptive statistics are generally more useful the greater the sample size; if the whole population is included you can have a far greater understanding of the attributes of the population. This is why many governments commission expensive and time-consuming censuses. Having data that cover the entire population gives you a very powerful tool for understanding that population (in theory at least, all censuses have flaws and often the biggest of these is that they do not include specific chunks of a population such as illegal immigrants or low-income workers[*]). If the sample includes the whole population, then descriptive statistics give us incredibly useful information that can be used to plan health services and allocate finite resources.

INFERENTIAL STATISTICS

Inferential statistics (also called inductive statistics) are used when it is impracticable to have all the data for a population you are interested in. This might be because of the size of the population – larger populations will be more difficult and costly to measure. It could be because of difficulties in making the appropriate measurements of a population – the time taken to collect data may mean these data are out of date by the time they are all collected. Or it could

---

[*] See, for example, US Government Accountability Office. *2010 Census: The Bureau's Plans for Reducing the Undercount Show Promise, but Key Uncertainties Remain*. GAO-08-1167T. Washington, DC: US Government Accountability Office; 2008. Available at: www.gao.gov/products/GAO-08-1167T (accessed 18 May 2013).

be because of the data being unavailable – for example, where you want to know the likely impact of a public health intervention before the programme is started, you will need to make some estimates based on indirect evidence. Inferential statistics can also be used to generate or test hypotheses about particular populations.

The basic premise of inferential statistics is that you are trying to *make conclusions based on the available data but those conclusions reach beyond what the data itself shows*.

An incredibly common use of statistics is in trying to understand what people think about a particular issue – an opinion poll. In an opinion poll a sample of people is used to try to gain an insight into what the whole population may feel about that issue. Similarly, in medical research sampling techniques are used in the design of studies to try to make sure that they are representative of the population of interest and therefore the results can be generalised to that population. Sampling techniques have to be robust and as free from bias as possible in order for the results to be genuinely useful and generalisable (*see* Chapter 4 for more on sampling techniques).

When inferential statistics are used we need to know how likely our results are to have occurred because of real effects of the variables we are studying rather than by chance. If a study suggests that a drug is effective in treating a particular disease, we need to know how likely it is that the experimental result is valid and accurately reflects the true effectiveness of that drug. This is where statistical significance can help us.

STATISTICAL SIGNIFICANCE

Statistical significance is a term that is commonly misused or misunderstood. It does not mean that a result has any importance, that it is meaningful or that it is a more accurate result than another result. *Statistical significance means that a result is **unlikely** to have arisen by chance alone*.

It is important to note that even if a result is *unlikely* to have occurred by chance, it may have done so. Unlikely events do occur – for example, phaeochromocytoma is unlikely to be the cause of high blood pressure but it has to be considered as a potential cause, particularly in those patients who have headaches, excessive sweating, anxiety, palpitations and weight loss. You are unlikely to diagnose a patient with a phaeochromocytoma but it is possible (the yearly incidence is two to eight per million. Knowing whether a result is meaningful and useful can only be fully understood by reviewing the initial research question, the way it has been tackled and how this may relate to your own patients. Reading the methods section of a paper should help in understanding whether a result is reasonable or answers the clinical questions you have (*see* Chapter 7 for more on how to translate clinical questions into answerable questions). This is one reason why having some understanding of research methodologies is useful even if you are never going to conduct your own research. Being able to comprehend the strengths and weaknesses of research can enable you to make better clinical decisions based on what you have read.

Remember that accuracy and significance are not the same. If we have a well-designed experiment that has effectively avoided bias as much as possible, so that the results are as accurate as possible, the results of that experiment are more likely to be accurate but they are not necessarily more likely to be significant. Whether the results are significant depends on there being a real relationship between the variables being measured.

THE NULL HYPOTHESIS AND P-VALUES

Q **2.6**   What is the significance level at which a result is generally taken to be significant?

a) 95%
b) 0.01
c) 1%
d) 0.5
e) 0.001

Q **2.7**   True or false?
a) The p-value needs to be set before an experiment is started.
b) The significance level should be set before an experiment is started.
c) The null hypothesis states that there is no relationship between the variables being studied.
d) A p-value represents the chance of obtaining a similar result if the study is repeated.
e) A p-value represents the chance that a result at least as extreme would occur by chance, given the null hypothesis being correct.
f) If the significance level is exceeded by a result this means that the null hypothesis is proven to be wrong.

Q **2.8**   Which of the following is the best definition of a type I error?
a) Falsely rejecting the null hypothesis when there is not a real relationship between the variables
b) Falsely rejecting the null hypothesis when there is a real relationship between the variables
c) Failing to reject the null hypothesis when there is not a relationship between the studied variables
d) That there is a relationship between the variables that is not demonstrated by the study
e) A false negative

The null hypothesis is often used to explain the idea of statistical significance; this is the hypothesis that *there is no relationship between variables*. The null hypothesis is rejected if a statistically significant result is found.

Commonly, the level at which a result is deemed to be significant is if that result would occur by chance less than one time in 20 (or a p-value of <0.05, or there being more than a 95% chance that the null hypothesis can be correctly rejected). This level is arbitrary; there is no particular mathematical reason why it is set at this level,* but any result that does not meet this criterion is normally considered to favour the null hypothesis – thereby suggesting that a relationship between the variables has not been found. Many authors consider a p-value of less than 0.01 to be highly significant.

It is very difficult to prove anything with certainty but we can much more easily show something to be false. Therefore, if the null hypothesis is rejected it is found incompatible with the result from a study. This is not the same as the null hypothesis itself being wrong, just that the study does not support it.

The definition of the p-value that you need to know is that it is *the chance of obtaining a result at least as extreme if the null hypothesis were true*. Therefore, if the p-value is <0.05 there is less than a 5% chance that the result of a study would have occurred if there was no relationship between the variables being studied. Note that the significance level should be set before the data are collected and if the p-value is less than the significance level then the null hypothesis is rejected. *The p-value is therefore not the same as the significance level.*

As an example of how this may be relevant to GPs, advocates of homeopathic remedies cite studies that show a benefit for people that use them, but there are meta-analyses that show homeopathy does not have any significant benefit.† One reason for this apparent paradox is that if you perform enough

---

* The statistician RA Fisher, in his seminal work *Statistical Methods for Research Workers* (1925), proposed that the p-value should be 0.05 as a minimum for a result to be considered statistically significant and this is now widely accepted.
† See Ernst E. Homeopathy: what does the 'best' evidence tell us? *Med J Aust.* 2010; **192**(8): 458–60.

studies you will expect a proportion of them to produce a result that falsely rejects the null hypothesis. This is known as a *type I error*, falsely rejecting the null hypothesis when there is not a relationship between the variables being studied. A meta-analysis pulls together the results of several studies. This can show more clearly whether there is a real relationship between variables and produce a more robust answer to a research question (*see* Chapter 5 for a discussion of meta-analysis).

A *type II error* is failing to reject the null hypothesis when it is actually false. This can be understood as a false negative, not finding a relationship between the variables being studied when there is one. A type I error, as described earlier, would conversely be seen as a false positive. Both type I and type II errors occur because a statistical test can return either false positives or false negatives.

HOW TO EVALUATE STATISTICS

Q 2.9 Which of the following is an expression of how likely a result from a study is to be consistently replicated in further studies?
a) Validity
b) Reliability
c) Precision
d) Accuracy

Q 2.10 If a study produces a measurement that is recorded to four decimal places, this is which of the following?
a) Valid
b) Reliable
c) Accurate
d) Precise

Q 2.11 If the same study is later found to have a systematic error in its measurement protocol, which of the following is not met?
a) Validity
b) Reliability
c) Accuracy
d) Precision

It is clear that statistics are most useful if we understand them and know how to evaluate them. There are some key concepts that help with evaluating statistics. These are reliability, precision, accuracy and validity. These are not uniquely used in statistical analysis but are used in different ways in other scientific study and there is some debate regarding their appropriate use. Probably the most useful are reliability and validity.

Reliability is an expression of how likely a result from a study is to be consistently replicated when another person or group undertakes a similar study. Precision is often used to mean the same as reliability. If you think of firing arrows at a target, if all our arrows are close together they demonstrate high precision, but they may not be grouped around the bull's eye.

Accuracy is how close those arrows are to the bull's eye – in a study this would be how close we are to measuring what we aimed to measure. A value may be expressed to several decimal places but this is unhelpful if the value is not very close to the target. Do not mistake higher precision for increased accuracy. *Validity is similar to accuracy but is also understood to be a wider evaluation of how well a study represents reality or measures what it set out to measure.*

If we are presented with a result from a study how should we evaluate it? If the result is closely replicated in several studies it is more *reliable* and therefore more likely to be helpful but we also want to know how *accurate, or valid,* the result is. This means, once again, going back to the methods section of a paper and understanding what is being measured and why. We also need to ask whether the result is useful for our day-to-day practice. Studies may confirm that a new anti-hyperglycaemic drug reduces HbA1c but this is only useful if it is also shown that patients live for longer with fewer complications of diabetes. What we need is *patient-oriented evidence, not disease-oriented evidence.*

Implicit in this need for patient-oriented evidence is that we need evidence that can change practice. This could be by providing us with an effective, safe new drug to help patients with specific conditions or by providing evidence that existing treatments should be used more cautiously because of side effects or adverse reactions or because patient outcomes are not often improved.

For example, there is some evidence that some statins are associated with an increased risk of diabetes.[*] However, the consensus remains that statins are useful treatments that prevent many avoidable deaths from cardiovascular disease. In order to fully understand the debate around such issues we have to be able to interpret the results of studies ourselves. This is something we consider further in Chapter 7.

LIMITATIONS OF STATISTICS

Healthcare is very expensive and it is becoming more so as the cost of new drugs increases, expectations rise, there is more chronic illness and people live longer. It is important that as GPs we use resources in a meaningful way – we

---

[*]   See, for example, Huupponen R, Viikari J. Statins and the risk of developing diabetes. *BMJ.* 2013; 346: f3156.

need to know how to treat our patients based on the best available evidence of what treatments are most effective and cost-effective.

We have to make decisions for our individual patients based on cost-effectiveness analysis for the whole community. In England and Wales this is one of the functions of the National Institute for Health and Care Excellence. As GPs we need to know how to access and interpret data on cost-effectiveness. We also need to know when to treat the individual patient in a manner that may not be considered to be appropriate for other patients.

There is a great deal of evidence that we will not have time to read and translate into our practice. This is why we need other methods of making decisions, including using meta-analyses and trusting expert opinion. We look in more depth at these issues in Chapters 7 and 8. For now, it is enough to recognise that evidence and statistics have limits in their usefulness.

CONCLUSION

It is evident that statistics and evidence can be and are misused. Statistics themselves do not tell us how we should act: they need to be interpreted and understood in a context. This context includes the original research problem and how that relates to patients, the economic context and the wider social, political and economic environment. Some subjects are also far more likely to be researched than others. This is why learning about research methods and statistics for the AKT should be seen as grounding for many aspects of your medical practice.

CHAPTER 3

Introduction to statistical methods

INTRODUCTION

In this chapter we will look at some of the building blocks of statistical methods such as averages and the normal distribution. We also look at graphical representation of data, choosing a statistical test and types of bias. These are all topics that are covered in the AKT, but they are also the basis for a more sophisticated use and understanding of data and statistics. First we need to consider how data can be classified into different types. Understanding that there are different types of data helps when deciding on appropriate ways to use and understand them.

Q 3.1 Choose the single best answer from the following options. Levels of measurement are:
a) different heights of data on a bar chart
b) basic techniques for measuring data
c) advanced statistical analysis tools
d) the hierarchy of data types
e) questions regarding how studies are performed.

Q 3.2 Choose the single best answer from the following options. Temperature as measured by the centigrade scale is a type of:
a) nominal data
b) ordinal data
c) interval data
d) ratio data.

Q 3.3   Choose the single best answer from the following options. Answers on a Likert scale from strongly dislike to strongly like are what type of data?
a) Nominal data
b) Ordinal data
c) Interval data
d) Ratio data

Q 3.4   Choose the single best answer from the following options. Data that consist of a list of names would be considered which level of measurement?
a) Nominal
b) Ordinal
c) Interval
d) Ratio

LEVELS OF MEASUREMENT

Data can be collected or produced in many different ways; the data collected vary in their attributes. This is important to understand, as it affects how data can be presented, manipulated and understood. There are statistical tests that make most sense with a particular type of data. For example, it makes less sense to talk of the average gender in a group of people than it does to talk about the average height of that group of people. The concept that there are different types of data is often referred to as 'levels of measurement'; this encompasses the idea that there is a hierarchy within data types, with some being more useful than others.

Nominal data

The simplest type of data is nominal data – this is simply data that are a name for something, such as nationality, gender or type of doctor. Essentially, nominal data are data that cannot meaningfully have a specific number attached to them. You may assign women the number 1 and men the number 2 for the purposes of data entry, but you could assign any number to either; it doesn't matter which number is assigned to a group, as long as each group has its own number. This means that nominal data cannot meaningfully have mathematical operations performed on them. It doesn't make sense to add or multiply names. The mode (the most common item) is the appropriate central tendency measure to describe nominal data.

Ordinal data

Ordinal data can be put into a meaningful order but the degree of difference between data points is not known. An example of ordinal data would be ranking of physicians' preferences for using different medications to treat a particular condition. The data are in order but you cannot tell what the difference is between data points – it cannot be measured meaningfully. A medication ranked the most popular cannot be said to be twice as good as a medication ranked second. It makes most sense to use the median (the middle-ranked item) as the measure of central tendency for ordinal data, but using the mode also makes sense. Using the mean makes less sense, because of the lack of a consistent difference between data points.

Interval and ratio data

Interval data have a fixed mathematical difference between each point. For example, temperature lies on an interval scale – the difference between 36°C and 37°C is the same as the difference between 37°C and 38°C. However, data in this category do not have a zero point where there is nothing that can be measured. A temperature of 0°C does not mean the absence of temperature but refers to the freezing point of water. The zero is an arbitrary point. You could equally imagine a useful and valid temperature scale that had zero as the freezing point of another chemical compound, such as carbon dioxide. Because the choice of the zero point is arbitrary, there are limits to the mathematical operations you can meaningfully do with interval data; you cannot meaningfully multiply interval data but you can add and subtract it.

Data that are part of a set that does have a definite zero point – for example, height or weight – are called *ratio data* or *scale data*. Interval or ratio data can be subject to more statistical tests and mathematical manipulation. Doubling height or weight does make sense.

It is possible to use the arithmetical mean as the measure of central tendency for interval and ratio data. It is also possible to measure the spread of the data using the range (the largest number minus the smallest number) and standard deviation (a measure of the average distance from the mean of a data set).

DESCRIPTIVE STATISTICS

Q 3.5 Match the following types of descriptive statistic with the most appropriate definition.

1) Median	a) The difference between the smallest and largest data point
2) Standard deviation	b) The arithmetical average
3) Range	c) The most common item of data
4) Mode	d) Data ranked in order and split into four sets, each with the same number of points
5) Mean	e) A measure of the spread of the data around the mean
6) Quartile	f) The middle point of the data when ranked in order

Q 3.6 Work out the mean, median, mode and range of the data presented in this table.

5	3	3	1
2	2	1	3
4	3	3	3
1	6	4	4

Mean	
Median	
Mode	
Range	

Measures of central tendency: the mean, median and mode

Measures of central tendency are useful in expressing what could be considered the midpoint or the typical value in a data set. However, as we have already seen, there are three commonly used ways of calculating this that apply in different situations.

If the average is mentioned, it often refers to the *mean – that is, the arithmetical average whereby every number is added together and then divided by how many numbers there are.* The big downside to the mean is that it can be misleading when there are outliers or a very skewed distribution. The mean for the data in Question 3.6 is 48/16 = 3

The median is the value that falls in the middle of the data set if all the values are put in order of size. This value is less affected by outliers than the mean. Because of this, the median is often used to describe skewed distributions. The median for Question 3.6 is 3. Note that where there is an even number of data values, you find the two numbers in the middle and then add these together and divide by 2.

The mode is the most frequently occurring value in a data set. It is not always a single value – bimodal distributions, for example, are characterised by two equally frequent modes. The mode's biggest advantage is that it can be used with non-numerical data – for example, the most commonly used drugs for a particular condition. The mode for the data in Question 3.6 is 3.

Measures of dispersion or spread: range, percentiles, quartiles and standard deviation

The range is the difference between the largest and smallest values in a data set. Therefore, it gives a good sense of the dispersion of the values – whether they are clustered closely together or spread out.

Percentiles (or centiles) are the number of data points divided by 100 with the data set out in order, normally from smallest to largest. They are useful in working out where a figure falls in a data set. If a data set includes 300 data points, then each centile includes three data values. If a value is found to be on the 20th centile, that means that 20% of the data points fall below that value.

Quartiles, however, are more useful for summarising data: they are the 25th centile (the lower quartile), the 50th centile (the median) and the 75th centile (the upper quartile). *The interquartile range is often used to show the middle 50% of the data between the 25th and 75th centiles.* The mean of this range can be more useful in estimating the central tendency of a data set where there are outliers.

The *standard deviation describes how much variation there is from the mean.* The larger the standard deviation the more spread out the data are. If the standard deviation is large, this may reflect a large degree of uncertainty in experimental results or it may reflect a heterogeneous (very different) sample or population. It is important to contemplate what this means in the context of research you are considering – look at what is being measured and why.

THE NORMAL DISTRIBUTION

Q 3.7 In a normal distribution, what proportion of data will fall within one standard deviation either side of the mean (to one decimal place)?
 a) 99.7%
 b) 95.4%
 c) 68.3%
 d) 34.2%

Q 3.8 True or false?
a) There is only one normal distribution, which is why it is called the normal distribution.
b) There are many normal distributions.
c) The normal distribution cannot be used to calculate deviation from the mean.
d) The normal distribution can be graphically represented by a bell curve.
e) Whether the data are normally distributed or not is not very important when choosing a statistical test.

Q 3.9 Choose one or more answers from the following options. In a normal distribution:
a) the data lies roughly equally on either side of the mean
b) the median has the same value as the mean
c) the mode has a higher value than the mean
d) the mode has a smaller value than the mean
e) the median has a smaller value than the mean

The idea of a normal (also called a Gaussian) distribution is very important to understand. Many statistical techniques are only appropriate when data are normally (or close to normally) distributed. It is a theoretical distribution that can be described as a bell-shaped curve that is symmetrical around the mean value of the sample or population. In a normal distribution, the median will be the same as the mean and the mode. *In a normal distribution, 68.3% of data will lie within one standard deviation either side of the mean, 95.4% within two standard deviations and 99.7% within three standard deviations.* A graph of three normal distributions is shown in Figure 3.1.

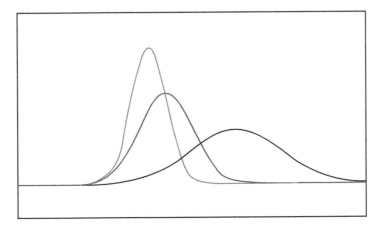

FIGURE 3.1 Three different but normally distributed data sets represented graphically

Note that there is not a single 'normal distribution'. The graph shows three different normal distributions, all of which fulfil the key criterion of being symmetrical around the mean. *The 'normal distribution' therefore includes the idea that data are symmetrically grouped around the mean in a bell shape* rather than a specific height and width of the graph. The width and height of the graph is determined by the standard deviation of the data, whereas the mean defines the centre of the curve.

Skewed distributions

Data with a longer tail to one side of the central measure when plotted are said to be skewed. Negative skew, also known as skew to the left, has a longer or fatter tail to the left side (smaller values) when graphed. Positive skew is the opposite, with a longer or fatter tail to the right side (higher values). In a negatively skewed distribution the mode will be greater than both the median and the mean. Likewise, in a positively skewed distribution the mode will be less than the median and the mean. It is frequently held that in a positively skewed data set, the mean is greater (or to the right on a graph) than the median, whereas in a negatively skewed data set the mean is less than the median. However, this rule is very often wrong when distributions are more complicated with evident asymmetry in the size of each tail or when there is more than one mode. Figure 3.2 provides graphs demonstrating simple skew:

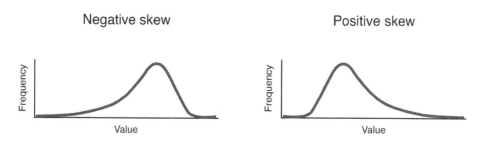

FIGURE 3.2 Example of **(a)** negative skew and **(b)** positive skew: in these simple cases of skew you would expect mean < median < mode in the negative skew and mean > median > mode in the positive skew

GRAPHICAL REPRESENTATION OF DATA

Q 3.10 Match the type of graph to the most appropriate definition.

   1) Pie chart   a) The length of bars is proportional to the values
                       they represent
   2) Bar chart   b) A two-dimensional plot of ordered observations
                       that are connected
   3) Histogram   c) Shows relative frequencies for a relatively small
                       selection of categories
   4) Line chart   d) Adjacent bars whose area matches the frequency of
                       observations in an interval

Q 3.11 True or false?
   a) Bar charts are useful for continuous (interval or ratio) data.
   b) Histograms are bar charts that use frequencies rather than percentages.
   c) Pie charts with many categories are easy to read.
   d) Line graphs are not suitable for continuous data.
   e) Histograms should only be used for continuous data.
   f) Scatter plots cannot have more than two variables.
   g) Box plots are a good way of comparing the median, range and inter-
      quartile range of variables.
   h) Frequency tables should always show relative frequencies.

Frequency tables, pie charts and bar charts are useful for presenting qualitative or categorical data (data that fit into categories rather than having a meaningful numerical value). Histograms, box plots, line graphs and scatter plots are useful for presenting quantitative or numerical data. Scatter plots are good for showing the relationship between two (or sometimes more than two) variables. Remember that simple presentation is nearly always more useful than any graphical effects. Be wary of three-dimensional graphs or graphs that use pictures to represent categories. These can be difficult to read and misrepresent the size of categories. Also be wary of charts with axes that do not start at zero or are logarithmic – these distort the differences between categories.

Frequency tables

These show the number in each category set out in a table – the frequency with which each category occurs. They may also include the relative frequency – that is, the proportion of the sample that falls into each category. The example outlined in Figure 3.3 sets out the frequencies of chronic diseases within a practice population. Note that the percentages here are not relative to one another, as the categories are not mutually exclusive (a patient could have diabetes, chronic kidney disease and ischaemic heart disease).

	Number of patients	Percentage of practice list
Diabetes	225	6%
Ischaemic heart disease	150	4%
Chronic kidney disease	123	3.3%
Stroke or transient ischaemic attack	68	1.8%

FIGURE 3.3 A simple frequency table showing the number of patients with certain chronic diseases in a practice of 3750 patients

Pie charts

These are very common and they are an easy and simple way to present relative frequencies when there are only a few categories that are mutually exclusive and so can be added up to make 100%. Each category is represented by a slice of the circle (or pie); the area in each slice is proportional to the relative frequency. They are often presented as three-dimensional, which is misleading because some slices will appear to have more area or volume than others. Also remember to look at the number as well as the percentage in each category – if the numbers in each category are small, the results have to be treated with caution. Pie charts, while commonly used, are not seen to be as useful as other

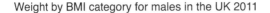

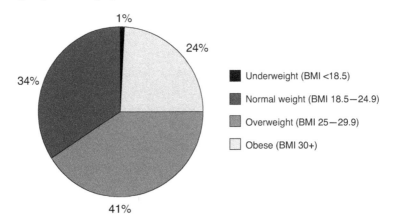

Weight by BMI category for males in the UK 2011

1%
24%
34%
41%

- Underweight (BMI <18.5)
- Normal weight (BMI 18.5–24.9)
- Overweight (BMI 25–29.9)
- Obese (BMI 30+)

FIGURE 3.4 A pie chart showing UK data for male weight in 2011 – the percentage labels have been added so it is easier to compare categories (data from Public Health England)

types of graph by many statisticians because research has shown that they are often misinterpreted. This is because pie charts use area rather than length for comparison and area is harder to judge than length. Thus pie charts are less helpful than bar charts for comparing categories with accuracy.

Bar charts

Bar charts are used to display the frequency of items in discrete categories of data or particular attributes, such as the mean value for a category. Bar charts are more helpful than pie charts in several ways, but particularly when there are a lot of categories to be presented. Typically, they present frequencies on the y-axis (the vertical axis) and categories on the x-axis (the horizontal axis), but switching this around can be useful when there are lots of categories or where they have long labels. The height (or length) of the bar represents the frequency of the result.

Similarly to pie charts, bar charts are best used for categorical data, but unlike pie charts the frequencies do not have to add up to 100%. When presenting nominal data, it does not matter in which order the bars are shown, but with ordinal data there is an inherent order that should be preserved. It is also possible to present data split into subgroups by grouping bars together or by stacking them on top of one another. They can also be used to compare data from different time points or after different interventions.

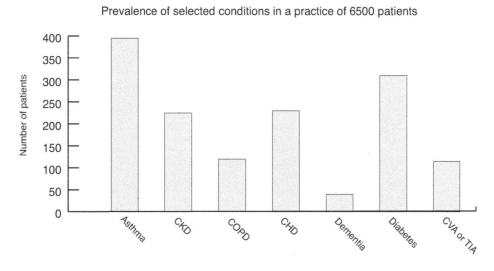

FIGURE 3.5 A bar chart with counts of patients in selected categories of chronic disease (CKD = chronic kidney disease, COPD = chronic obstructive pulmonary disease, CHD = coronary heart disease, CVA = cerebrovascular accident, TIA = transient ischaemic attack)

Bar charts can distort data if they are not comparing like with like or have graphic effects such as three-dimensional bars. A common distortion is to start the axis at a value other than zero, which makes the ratio of categories appear very different to reality. Also beware scales that have any transformation, such as logarithmic scales – these can distort differences between categories. Figure 3.5 shows an example of a bar chart.

Histograms

Histograms are used to display continuous data such as interval and ratio data. They show the shape of the distribution of the data. In a histogram, continuous data are split into ranges known as bins. The area of a bar represents the number of data points falling within that range. When reading a histogram, pay careful attention to the ranges chosen – the width of the bars should be equal where the ranges are equal. The bins should touch one another because the data are continuous. If a bin does not contain any values, then there should be a gap between bars – that is, the bar is shown as having zero height. Look at the shape to see if the data are clustered around the mean or skewed and also look for outliers or gaps in the data. Outliers will affect the mean, the range and the standard deviation of a data set. It is likely that gaps will have a similar impact.

Note that histograms differ from bar charts in that they show the distribution of data within ranges whereas bar charts compare the frequency of variables. Bar charts normally plot categorical data (data that can be sorted into

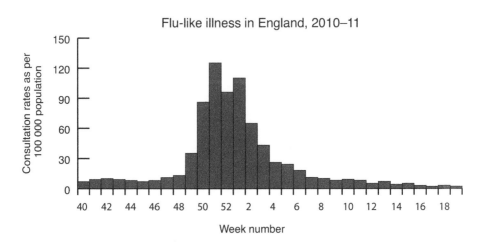

FIGURE 3.6 A histogram showing flu-like illness consultation rates in England in 2010–11: note the bars are adjacent to one another, as the data are continuous; also note the dip over the Christmas week (52), probably due to data collection difficulties rather than a real drop in illness rates (data from Public Health England)

mutually exclusive categories); histograms can only plot continuous data. The bars in bar charts can often be rearranged without it making any difference to the meaning of the graph but this is not the case for a histogram. Figure 3.6 gives an example of a histogram.

Line graphs

Line graphs are also used to show continuous data. They are often used to show time series data, which plot changes in one or more variables over time. They are useful for identifying patterns over time, such as seasonal variation in disease activity. They can also be used for other continuous data series such as distance – for example, showing how distance from a source of pollution affects asthma rates. The data need to be collected sufficiently often to make meaningful comparison possible and to ensure that important variations are not omitted.

The x-axis should represent the continuous variable, such as time or distance, and the y-axis should indicate the measurement. Where several data series are collected, they can be shown together to allow easy comparison of trends. Line graphs should not be used for categorical data – that cannot be joined meaningfully. A common use of line graphs in biostatistics is a Kaplan–Meier survival curve, which shows the proportion of people surviving after diagnosis or treatment.

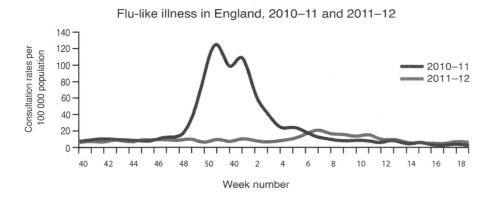

FIGURE 3.7 A line graph of the same data as shown in Figure 3.6, with additional data for 2011–12: each year is shown as a separate line, which makes the graph much easier to read than if a histogram were used (data from Public Health England)

Box plots

Often called a box-and-whisker plot, this is used to show the distribution of interval data with the central value and variability also shown. There is a central box with a line across it to represent the median, the edges of the box represent the upper and lower quartiles, and lines (whiskers) extend from the box to the maximum and minimum values. This can show any skew in the distribution and suggest whether there are outliers. They are useful when comparing two or more data sets. For example, they could be used to compare the effect of a drug in men and women or cholesterol levels before and after an intervention.

Box plots can be drawn either vertically or horizontally, although the former is more common. The whiskers can be used to represent values other than maximum and minimum, so make sure you check what is being shown. Some plots include outliers as dots beyond the extent of the whiskers. The size of the box is sometimes used to show the relative size of each group being graphed, with the height (if the box is shown horizontally) or width (if the box is shown vertically) proportional to the size of the group.

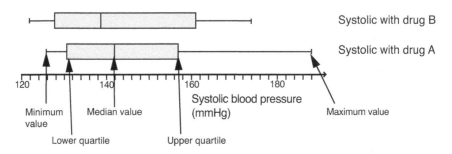

FIGURE 3.8 A box plot showing the difference in systolic blood pressure with two anti-hypertensive medications (labels added to show the values used to construct the plot)

Scatter plots

'Bivariate' data have two quantitative variables for each measurement – for example, age and height of study participants. It is often easier to interpret bivariate data if the data are graphed. A scatter plot maintains the relationship of the two variables, with one on the y-axis and the other on the x-axis.

If there is a relationship between the variables it is possible to see both the strength of the relationship (how closely the points cluster together or along a line) and the direction of the relationship. If the variables increase together it is a positive association, or if one decreases as the other increases this is a negative association. Note that the line of association does not have to be straight – it is often curved. For example, in a graph showing mortality against time from diagnosis for a terminal disease, the line tends to be curved, with a small proportion of patients living longer than most others.

It is possible to use a scatter plot to graph more than two variables through the use of three-dimensional charts and gradated colours. These charts can be more difficult to read unless carefully constructed. Figure 3.9 gives an example of a simple scatter plot.

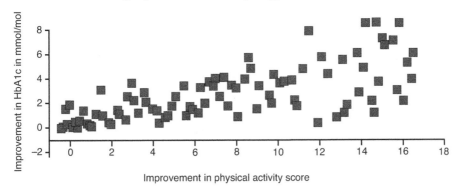

FIGURE 3.9 A scatter plot of changes in HbA1c with changes in physical activity scores (this is based on the well-known relationship between diabetic control and physical exercise, but the figures are not from a real study)

CORRELATION

Q 3.12 From the following options, choose all answers that could be true. A correlation coefficient of +1 implies:
a) there is a perfect correlation between two variables
b) there may be falsification of results as there appears to be no error in measurements
c) as one variable increases, the other variable decreases
d) as one variable increases, the other variable also increases
e) when graphed the relationship would be shown by a straight line, with all points falling on it

Q 3.13 Which of the following is the best definition of a confounding variable?
a) A variable that is related to both the dependent and independent variables being studied and which alters both.
b) A variable that causes the independent variable to alter without an obvious cause.
c) A factor that has not been accounted for in the design of a study.
d) A variable that causes results to be confusing.
e) A variable that has been studied but its behaviour is unknown.

Correlation is a measure of the extent to which one variable changes as another variable changes. If correlation is positive, this means both variables change in the same direction – for example, as air pollution increases so does the prevalence of asthma. Negative correlation means that as one variable increases the other decreases – for example, as age increases, kidney function decreases. If there is correlation this does not mean that every study participant demonstrates the same relationship between variables, just that there is a tendency for one variable to change in a particular direction as the other variable changes.

Spurious correlation is where there wrongly appears to be a correlation between two variables because of another factor that is linked to both of them. The third factor here would be referred to as a confounder. If a study shows a link between poor oral health and oesophageal cancer rates, you may postulate that there is a link between the two; in fact, smoking is a causative factor in both and is therefore a confounding variable. Correlations can also appear to exist, even when there is no real relationship between variables, because of chance or poor methodology.

If you consider a scatter plot, the closer the points are to the line of association then the higher the correlation between the variables. Correlation is often measured using Pearson's product-moment correlation coefficient or Spearman's rank correlation coefficient (*see* Figure 3.10).

Pearson's product-moment correlation coefficient is only appropriate for data that show a linear relationship, in that the data falls on or around a straight line when plotted. Spearman's rank correlation coefficient does not have the same requirement, so it can be used with data that fall on a curved line. It is always worth examining the graphical representation of the data, because there are several ways in which a data set can have the same correlation coefficient and only one of those is a linear relationship.[*]

The more closely the relationships alter with each other, the nearer the (Pearson's) correlation coefficient will be to 1, either +1 for a positive relationship or –1 for a negative relationship. A correlation of 1 means that all points lie on the same line, but this would be unusual because there is normally some error in the measurement of variables. Note that Spearman's rank correlation coefficient gives a result of +1 when as one variable increases the other *always* increases, and it gives a result of –1 when as one variable increases the other *always* decreases.

Remember that correlation does not mean that there is a causal relationship between variables. However, in some cases, such as height compared with age in children, it is obvious that as average age increases so will average height,

---

[*] Anscombe's quartet illustrates how different relationships can have the same correlation coefficient and the same summary statistics (mean and variance). See Anscombe FJ. Graphs in statistical analysis. *Am Stat.* 1973, **27**(1): 17–21.

and so correlation can be taken to imply causation. Further investigation, such as completing a randomised controlled trial, is often necessary to prove causal links after correlation is found. Causality can be established if a relationship is shown that has a time order, a positive dose–effect relationship and there are not any confounding factors. Internal validity is *the degree to which it can be shown that there is a causal relationship between variables.*

CONFIDENCE INTERVALS

Q 3.14 Which of the following options will help a confidence interval become narrower? Choose one or more answers.
a) A smaller sample size
b) A significantly increased sample size
c) Studying a population with a lot of variability
d) Studying a population with more homogeneity
e) Having a more complex study design

A confidence interval is an estimate of the range of values within which the true parameter lies. A parameter applies to the whole population and not just the sample being studied. Knowing the confidence interval is necessary, because a sample is highly likely to vary in some ways from the population from which it is drawn.

The confidence interval is calculated from the observations in a study. It is based on the idea that if you drew lots of samples from the population being studied, you would be able to combine the results to get closer to the actual parameter. A confidence interval is not the probability of a particular result being the true parameter for the population. It is a range within which the population parameter can be expected to be found in a proportion of samples. This proportion is commonly set at 95%. If a confidence interval of 99% is used, then the true population parameter is 99% likely to fall within that range.

This is similar and related to the idea of the level of significance (or a p-value) discussed in Chapter 5, but do not confuse the two definitions. The p-value signifies the probability that the result of a repeat of the trial or measurement would be equal to or more extreme than the one observed, if the null hypothesis was true (*see* Chapter 5).

Generally, the larger the sample size and the less variability (i.e. more homogeneity) within the population as a whole, then the smaller the confidence interval will be. If you study only a handful of subjects from within a very large population, there is a very good chance that they will vary significantly from the population as a whole, particularly if that population has a lot of variation within it, and this will lead to a wide confidence interval. More complex study designs generally increase the confidence interval. Where confidence intervals are very large this suggests that further, larger studies are necessary before any conclusions should be drawn. We will look further at confidence intervals when we consider relative risk and odds ratios in Chapter 5, including where the confidence interval crosses the line of no effect – meaning that the study has not found a significant difference between parameters.

PARAMETRIC AND NON-PARAMETRIC TESTS

Q 3.15 Which of the following are characteristics of non-parametric tests?
a) They make more assumptions about a population.
b) They assume that the population being studied fits into a normal distribution.
c) They are often simpler to use and interpret than parametric tests.
d) They are more powerful than parametric tests.
e) They do not rely on accurate sampling for their validity.

Parameters are values that describe a complete population – as opposed to a statistic, which is a value calculated from a sample. For example, the mean is a parameter when it is calculated for the whole population and a statistic when it is calculated from a sample. Why is this distinction important? Knowing the difference helps in understanding the difference between parametric and non-parametric tests.

Parametric methods are those statistical methods that are used when we know that the population we are studying fits into a normal or a related distribution. Non-parametric methods are those that do not assume that the population studied fits into a particular distribution.

As non-parametric tests make fewer assumptions about the population, they can be much more widely applied than parametric tests, and they are often simpler to use and interpret as well. However, when we would like to infer something about a population, a parametric test is more useful. Parametric tests are also more useful for more complicated modelling. If assumptions are incorrect, parametric tests can give misleading results, but if the assumptions are correct, then they can provide more accurate and precise statistics.

CHOOSING A TEST

A common practice question for the AKT relates to which tests should be used when. This is problematic: statisticians research and debate the circumstances under which certain tests can be appropriately used. Statistics is not a monolithic subject with only one right way to do things; it is evolving. There are reasons why tests should or should not be used in particular circumstances. The understanding, refinement and rejection of these reasons evolve in the same way as any other scientific subject.

Figure 3.10 has *suggestions* for the most appropriate tests in particular circumstances. It should be used with caution. It does not assume that these are rules written in stone. For example, there are good reasons why ordinal data could be treated in a similar way to interval data. Having a basic understanding of which tests may be applied in particular circumstances is often useful when reading research reports. However, it is advisable to discuss with an expert statistician if you need to choose a test for research purposes.

		Dependent variable			
		Nominal	Ordinal	Interval, normally distributed	Interval, non-normally distributed
Independent variable	Nominal	Chi-square test	Mann–Whitney U test	Student's t-test	Mann–Whitney U test
	Ordinal	Mann–Whitney U test	Spearman's rank correlation coefficient	Spearman's rank correlation coefficient and linear regression	Spearman's rank correlation coefficient
	Interval, normally distributed	Logistic regression		Pearson's product-moment correlation coefficient and linear regression	Linear regression
	Interval, non-normally distributed	Logistic regression		Pearson's product-moment correlation coefficient or Spearman's rank correlation coefficient and linear regression	Pearson's product-moment correlation coefficient or Spearman's rank correlation coefficient

FIGURE 3.10 Choice of statistical test, based on the level of measurement of the independent and dependent variables

Figure 3.10 uses the levels of measurement discussed at the beginning of this chapter. Note that interval-level data are split into normally distributed and non-normally distributed – that is, parametric and non-parametric. Figure 3.10 splits variables up into independent and dependent variables. The independent variable is also known as the explanatory variable, because changes in it explain changes in the dependent variable.

Here is a brief explanation of each of these tests. Remember that there are variations on many of these tests and also that there are many other tests that we have not mentioned.

Chi-squared test

This is used to compare observed data with an expected outcome. Expected means according to the null hypothesis – the proportions would be expected to be the same in two groups if there was no effect of a variable. This is a non-parametric test for nominal data. You may use it to compare groups – for example, smokers and non-smokers.

Mann–Whitney U test

This is a non-parametric test used to investigate whether differences in the median results for two groups could have occurred by chance. This applies to ordinal data so could be used when patients use a rating scale for pain or depression and are subject to different interventions.

Student's t-test

This is named after the pseudonym adopted by a statistician in a seminal paper, not because it is the favoured test of undergraduates! It is used to test whether the mean value in the dependent variable is the same for each of two groups. This is the parametric equivalent of the Mann–Whitney U test.

There is a paired version of this test, which tests whether the mean scores for a single group vary significantly under two different conditions. The data are paired – that is, there are two results for each research participant. This is useful when you compare results for a group, pre and post exposure to a drug or intervention.

Spearman's rank correlation coefficient

This was discussed briefly in the section on correlation earlier. It is used with ordinal data or with interval data that are put into rank order. It results in a correlation coefficient between -1 and $+1$. No correlation between the variables would result in a value of 0. An example of where this may be used is to look at how depression scores change, or not, in relationship to levels of exercise.

Pearson's product-moment correlation coefficient

This was also discussed in the section on correlation earlier. This is often referred to simply as the correlation coefficient. It is a parametric test that is used when both variables are interval-level data. It gives a figure for how strong the relationship is between the two variables. This is normally used with linear regression: in effect it is a measure of the linear correlation between the variables.

Linear regression

Used when you have two interval-level variables whereby you have two readings for each research participant. A simple example would be where calorie intake and weight change were measured and the strength of the relationship between increased calorie intake and weight gain can be seen. Typically, you would plot the points on a scatter plot and fit them with a line of regression to show the strength of the relationship. This can be used for more than two variables, which is called multiple linear regression.

Logistic regression

Used when the dependent variable is nominal with two values, such as yes or no. This is similar to linear regression except that the dependent variable is nominal rather than interval data. Like linear regression, it is possible to do multiple logistic regression when you have more than one independent variable. This could be used to investigate the link between having a heart attack (the nominal variable – yes or no) and blood pressure readings or cholesterol values.

BIAS

Bias is commonly used to suggest that a particular opinion is held with a refusal to contemplate the possible merits of alternative views. It has a related but more specific meaning in statistics; namely, that there *is a systematic distortion of results due to factors that have not been allowed for in designing, carrying out and reporting a study*. Figure 3.11 lists some different types of bias in statistics; it is possible for a study to have several types of bias. The aim of a good study is to try to avoid or reduce bias in order for the results to be more helpful, robust and generalisable.

Types of bias	
Systematic bias	External influences that may affect the accuracy of measurements and favour one outcome over another, such as where researchers are under pressure to produce a particular result.
Funding bias	Where a source of funding may affect the way the study is conducted and reported, such as drug company sponsorship of a study.
Selection bias	An error in choosing, or randomising, the individuals to take part in a study, whereby some groups or individuals are more likely to be chosen than others. This may occur when rigorous selection methods are not used.
Sampling bias	The research subjects are not representative of the population being considered. This is quite common when drugs are tested on young fit people rather than elderly patients with multiple morbidities.
Procedure bias	Where subjects in different groups are not treated the same, sometimes because of the group they are in. For example, being offered extra treatments because it is known they are being given an older drug or a placebo – this is why double-blinding is important.
Recall bias	Where research subjects are asked to recall events but do so inaccurately because of the inherent problems with relying on memory.
Lead-time bias	If a disease is discovered in a research subject at an earlier stage than other subjects, this makes it look like they have an increased survival over a set period of time. This can apply to screening programmes that appear to increase survival simply because people are detected at an earlier stage – the actual age at death may not be affected.
Late-look bias	Where information is gathered inappropriately late, meaning that some subjects cannot respond – this is particularly problematic when studying fatal diseases.
Spectrum bias	Evaluating a diagnostic test in a biased group of patients leading to an overestimate of the sensitivity and specificity of the test and therefore making the test appear more helpful than it really is. This may occur if the test is evaluated on a preselected group such as hospital patients rather than primary care patients or the general population.
Reporting or publication bias	If data are not reported there will be a skew in the data that is available and this can make an intervention look more or less useful than it really is. The obvious example would be withholding negative findings because it is felt they are not useful or interesting, or more problematically that they make a drug less likely to sell well.
Hawthorne effect	Where research subjects modify their behaviour because they know they are being studied. This is due to research participants', not researchers', expectations. An example may be that research participants wish to appear healthier than they really are and so do more exercise than normal and eat more healthily while being studied. There is evidence that this effect wears off after the study has been going for a week or so.
Pygmalion (or Rosenthal) effect	Where beliefs held by researchers encourage research participants to perform better than expected. This may be a particular problem with some psychological studies. If the researchers let the participants know that their performance is expected to improve if they receive a particular intervention, that knowledge may spur them on to achieve more than they would otherwise.
Golem effect	The opposite of the Pygmalion effect, where expectations are lowered so the participants do worse than they would have otherwise achieved.

FIGURE 3.11 Types of bias

CHAPTER 4

Qualitative methods

INTRODUCTION

Qualitative methods are often seen as less useful or less powerful than quantitative methods. They come lower in the hierarchy of evidence (*see* Chapter 5) and are often considered to deliver less robust evidence. They do, however, provide a different type of evidence, which may be as powerful, or more powerful, than that from quantitative methods, depending on what you want to know. *Qualitative research is about understanding the experiences of individuals or small groups.*

Statistical results from drug trials are important but they do not tell us how an *individual* will respond to a drug. As GPs we are constantly trying to understand the experiences of our patients. This is where qualitative methods are useful – they help to gain a deeper insight into the experiences of individuals and small groups.

Although research methods are split into quantitative and qualitative approaches, it is to some extent a false dichotomy. These methods can, and often do, inform and strengthen each other. Qualitative studies often use quantitative techniques to analyse data – for example, the average age and the range of ages of study participants. Like all methodologies, the usefulness of the research findings is based on how good a study is and how reliable the gathered information is.

The choice of methods should be based on what is being investigated and why, as well as what the results may be used for. Clearly, looking into the effectiveness of a drug is best done by a large randomised controlled study or meta-analysis. However, looking at how that drug affects people's lives is best done through interviews, questionnaires or other qualitative methods.

Be aware that when human behaviour is being studied, there is normally a theoretical standpoint that is used to interpret what is seen. Different groups of people view the world and interpret what they find and see in different ways. Indeed, this is true of researchers as much as, if not more than, other people. This is not unique to qualitative research: it is often argued that scientists can have worldviews that affect how they perform their experiments or research.

Much of the information we use as GPs is based on what we have learnt about treatments from our patients. Formalising that information and testing it for generalisability (that is, how well the results can be applied to people beyond those in the study) is helpful and what distinguishes research from anecdotal evidence. Conducting good qualitative research is difficult and calls for methods that minimise bias and get as close to the truth as possible.

Q 4.1 Qualitative research seeks to analyse the _____ people attribute to their _____ and circumstances. Which of the following suggestions fill in the gaps best?
a) data, research
b) data, experiences
c) associations, lives
d) experience, meanings
e) meanings, experiences

Q 4.2 Which of the following methods are commonly associated with qualitative research? There is one or more correct answer/s.
a) Grounded theory
b) Interviewing
c) Focus groups
d) Delphi technique
e) Statistical analysis
f) Experiments

Q 4.3 _____ refers to using more than one research method to help strengthen the conclusions from qualitative research. Which of the following terms fits best in the gap?
a) Triangulation
b) Saturation
c) Delphi technique
d) Experimenting
e) Purposive sampling

Q **4.4** What is it called when there is no longer any need to sample more people to reach new conclusions or to back up or challenge existing conclusions?
 a) Triangulation
 b) Saturation
 c) Delphi technique
 d) Experimenting
 e) Purposive sampling

PILOT STUDIES

A pilot study is a small study often completed before a bigger, more costly study. The aim is to evaluate feasibility, test and refine data collection methods, measure costs, discover adverse effects and decide whether a full-scale study is appropriate. In quantitative research, pilot studies are also used both to estimate how big the sample needs to be in order for the results to be as accurate as needed and to make an estimate of effect size.

Pilot studies are very common in qualitative research, as the data collection techniques often need to be refined before being applied in larger research projects. It is necessary to make sure they capture the data that they are intended to in a form that is useful and can be used to answer the research question. Pilot studies can highlight previously unconsidered circumstances that need to be reflected on before large-scale data collection can begin, such as restrictions on access to the population of interest. An example of an outcome of a pilot study would be that an interview schedule, when tested, is found to have too much ambiguity or allows too much freedom to researchers so that they do not collect comparable data. More positively, pilot studies may collect data that act as a stimulus to further research and raise new research questions.

TRIANGULATION

Combining methods can improve our knowledge more than using just a single method. Using a second method can help confirm or refute what has been found and is called triangulation. This is analogous to triangulation in trigonometry, where the location of an unknown point is determined by measuring distance and angles from known points. A single method can often give a good overview of a particular research subject, but using two or more methods can increase insights.

Triangulation can be utilised for qualitative, quantitative and mixed research, but it is most commonly used in qualitative studies. The basic premise is that research findings are strengthened if different methods lead to similar conclusions. For example, conducting focus groups around health concerns may bring up a list of problems that can be explored in structured interviews to acquire more detail and to test hypotheses. Some people may not feel comfortable in focus groups or interviews, so adding in anonymous questionnaires may add to the information already gathered.

Triangulation can be carried out by having more than one observer as well as having more than one method – obviously, if two or more independent observers reach similar conclusions then the results are more likely to be valid. Qualitative research often needs a theoretical underpinning to enable interpretation of the phenomena under investigation. Therefore, comparing the understanding of phenomena from different theoretical positions may also be helpful. We look at some common theoretical approaches later in this chapter.

SAMPLING METHODS AND SATURATION

Q 4.5   If every member of a population has an equal chance of being selected for a research project, what is this called?
a) Snowball sampling
b) Random sampling
c) Quota sampling
d) Stratified sampling
e) Grab sampling

Q 4.6   If a researcher uses participants to identify further people to take part in the research, what is this called?
a) Snowball sampling
b) Random sampling
c) Quota sampling
d) Stratified sampling
e) Grab sampling

Qualitative research needs to be robust in order to be applicable beyond the sample studied. It is important to target the appropriate research participants for the specific research question being asked. When a research project is designed, possible sources of bias, including sampling, need to be considered. Sampling a population makes research more manageable and more cost-effective than trying to study the whole population.

A number of sampling techniques have been developed to enable researchers to find the right research participants by aiming to get an appropriate cross-section of research participants. Here we look at some of the techniques that are commonly used.

Simple random sampling

In quantitative research, samples should be selected randomly to ensure the conclusions are robust and applicable to the population as well as the sample. Random sampling can also be used in qualitative research. For example, if the population you are interested in is the patients registered at a particular GP surgery, you may use random number tables (or a computer program) to pick out a sample from a list of all the patients at that surgery by using a numerical identifier, such as their patient numbers. This type of sampling is called *simple random sampling*. There is a risk that such a sample does not reflect the population in certain attributes such as age or gender and so other sampling methods have been developed, including stratified, quota and cluster sampling.

Stratified sampling

Sometimes it is desirable to have research participants with particular attributes. For example, if you are studying how social inclusion improves the health of elderly people, you will need a sample consisting of elderly people but you may also want those people to be drawn from different social or geographical environments.

Splitting the population into subgroups with similar characteristics and taking a sample that includes members from all subgroups is known as stratified sampling. This is used when subgroups vary from the overall population in some way. For example, the most obvious variation might be age or gender. These would both affect how people behave and you may want to consider how behaviour varies between groups or get an overall picture of how the population behaves.

All strata in this technique must be mutually exclusive – each and every person should be assigned to a single stratum. The strata should also be as homogeneous as possible, with well-defined criteria, and the differences between strata should be as large as possible.

Quota sampling

This is similar to stratified sampling in that the population is split into subgroups. The difference is that quotas are set. For example, 200 men and 200 women or 100 people in each 10-year age group from 16 to 66. There may be several quotas that are not mutually exclusive, such as gender and age; therefore, an individual may meet the criteria for two or more quotas. It is likely that the sample taken will be considerably larger than the largest quota, because all the quotas have to be met. This is often used when the views or experiences of particular segments of a population are sought.

The main drawback with quota sampling is that it is a non-probability technique, meaning it is not random, so there is a greater chance that some people will be selected than others. This means that this type of sample *may not* enable robust statistical results. Qualitative research is not looking for robust statistics and it is often more important to get an appropriate range of voices.

Cluster sampling

If the population is large, it sometimes helps to split it into groups and then sample from within those groups. These could be based on geographical location or on periods of time (such as how long someone has been on a particular drug). Once the population is split into groups (clusters), those groups can be sampled. Clustering is often used when the costs of a random sample of the whole population would be prohibitive.

Cluster sampling is often multistage, where the population is split into groups and then there is a further selection of groups from within the first set. It is possible for this to happen several times before individuals are selected for the sample. A good example would be using geographical data first to select several counties, then to select districts from those counties, and finally to select electoral wards before selecting individuals to be surveyed.

Opportunity sampling

There are several names for this type of sampling, such as accidental or grab sampling, but they all point towards the fact that individuals are selected through convenience. The sample may be selected based on a list of people known to have particular traits, such as a particular disease, and are selected without any randomisation. This is inevitable if there are only a small number of people in the population with that disease. The results can be helpful in understanding how people cope with a particular disease, such as the psychological effects of having a rare skin condition. Obviously this is a non-probability sampling technique that does not allow for robust inductive statistical analysis.

A variation on this is *snowballing*, where initial contact is made with an individual or group and associates of that individual or group are also asked to take part in the research, sometimes by the researcher and sometimes they are recruited by the research participants themselves. This is particularly useful for finding members of hidden, difficult-to-find or illegal populations. This may be the case, for example, when looking for homeless people or drug users to investigate aspects of their healthcare needs.

This type of sampling can give very misleading results if not treated with care. It is likely that people sampled in this way may not reflect the whole population in a variety of ways. People who are happier to be interviewed, for example, may have different characteristics, such as an outgoing personality or a particular subject they are keen to discuss. If you consider interviews being conducted on a busy shopping street, you will realise that there are several sources of bias – you miss a great number of people: those who do not shop in that area or who cannot get out to shop; those who cannot shop at that time; those who do not want to be interviewed because they are busy – workers on their lunch break or parents looking after fractious children.

The message is to understand how the sample was achieved and why. Be wary of any statistical inferences from non-random samples. Be aware of the limitations of research evidence with poor sampling techniques.

Saturation

Saturation is the idea that enough individuals have been sampled and enough data have been collected. In statistical research there are formulas to work out appropriate sample sizes. In qualitative research it is often difficult to know when enough people have been sampled to give reasonable and useful conclusions. If the research is a case study, then the sample may only be one person. If, however, the research needs a bigger sample, how can a researcher be sure that enough people have been included in the study?

There are several theoretical ideas regarding saturation, with no universally accepted methods of establishing saturation. *Saturation may be reached when no new data are collected over a predetermined number of interviews.* Alternatively, *saturation may be reached when no more study participants can be found without taking up considerable resources.* The aims of a study may determine when saturation is reached, with a more tightly focused study needing fewer participants. Factors affecting saturation may include the overall heterogeneity of the population; the types of data collection methods and the number of data collection methods used; the budget of the study; the intensity with which participants are studied; and the selection criteria used to select participants.

QUALITATIVE RESEARCH METHODOLOGY

Q 4.7 What does methodology refer to? Choose the best definition from the following options.
a) The system of methods, principles and rules used to undertake research
b) The study of the nature of being and existence
c) The justification for choosing particular research methods
d) The study of knowledge that aims to separate justified knowledge from opinion
e) The techniques chosen to answer a research question

Q 4.8 True or false?
a) Action research aims to solve a problem.
b) Grounded theory ensures researchers do not forget the theoretical underpinnings of their research.
c) Ethnography always involves living with a group of people to understand their culture.
d) Phenomenology aims to understand the meanings behind significant statements of research participants.
e) Phenomenology means identifying phenomena and then studying them via focus groups.

There are many different research approaches (or methodologies) in qualitative research. Having a basic understanding of some of these is helpful in understanding research results. There are a couple of important terms to understand first: epistemology and methodology.

Epistemology is the study of what can be known in terms of which beliefs can be justified and which are simply opinion. This is particularly important in qualitative research, because it is clear that the way people behave and react varies between cultures and within cultures. Researchers will have an epistemological framework that forms the theoretical base with which they approach their research in order to understand those cultures.

Methodology is the methods, principles and rules that are used in undertaking research. This is more than just the research methods. Methodology is about how epistemology and theoretical underpinnings are applied to answer a research question. Research methods are the interviews or focus groups and other techniques that are used to collect data. We look at a few qualitative research methods in the next section.

The theoretical underpinnings of qualitative research develop from epistemological stances. There are many theoretical frameworks that guide qualitative researchers and they are often nuanced. The most important of these theoretical underpinnings could be considered to be positivism, constructionism and pragmatism.

Objectivism holds that there is an objective truth that can be discovered by looking at the world around us. Objectivism is related to positivism. Positivist research often uses quantitative methods, because researchers want to measure things that can lead to knowing that objective truth.

Constructionism holds that truth is actually socially constructed. It is not possible to find a single truth because people interpret things through their previous experiences and dialogue with people around them.

Pragmatism suggests that we reach understanding through what works at the time, with reference to the ideas of others around us. The important thing for pragmatist research is to get to a useful answer. To do this, it is reasonable to draw on anything that helps.

Ethnography

Ethnography is literally 'writing of culture'; it is the systematic study of a social group or culture. It aims for depth of understanding with a lot of detail, sometimes referred to as 'thick description'. The methods used would include observation and participant observation and possibly interviews. There may also be documentary analysis. This research should be undertaken in the naturally occurring setting of the study subjects; therefore, the researcher undertakes fieldwork. The research should be conducted 'reflexively'. This means the impact of the researcher on the subjects is considered and explicitly addressed. The study outcomes could include descriptions of social interactions, behaviours and the perceptions that people within a particular group develop and share.

Ethnography may be considered to be analogous to documentary making – focusing on one subject and aiming to construct a coherent narrative about that subject. However, the difference is that ethnographers aim to construct the narrative from the viewpoint of the studied subject. The narrative should be allowed to emerge from the research subject rather than be imposed. The inherent difficulty here relates to the authority of the researcher to construct that narrative, especially when the culture the researcher is studying is not his or her own.

Grounded theory

Grounded theory is often contrasted to other social science research techniques, which, it could be argued, apply theory to the data. *Grounded theory tries to avoid preconceived ideas and instead allow theories to develop from the research data.* The data should be as free from bias as possible and the data should not have theory imposed before they are collected. The researcher will try to understand what the research participants perceive as significant. To do this, as data are collected, they are analysed to identify recurring themes that are assigned to categories. Once these categories are identified there will be further exploration to try to refine them. Eventually, a theoretical framework is constructed by integrating the categories into a single narrative.

The most common technique for research using grounded theory is probably in-depth interviews, but observation and focus groups may also be used. There is a wide variety of research that is conducted with some adherence to grounded theory and this is reflected in a diversity of research methods and outcomes.

Grounded theory can be useful when there has been little previous exploration of a particular research setting, so there is a limited amount of knowledge and theory about the research subjects or context. It can also be helpful when trying to discover the true concerns of a social group in order to target appropriate interventions. An example may be trying to understand what the health needs are of new migrants and how their own cultural beliefs interact with the cultural beliefs of their adopted home.

Phenomenology

Phenomenology is the study of subjective experience. As a research method this means trying to understand the different ways that people think about something. Research from this perspective holds that people have different ways of understanding the world and that even the way we experience the world varies. The language and discourse around an area of study will influence how phenomena are understood; language is a large part of the construction of the world of the research participants. Often research from a phenomenological perspective will look for significant statements from research participants and then explore the meaning that they give to those statements.

The methods that may be used in phenomenological research include participant observation and interviews. The aim is to explore the motivations and the perceptions of the research participants and investigate them in depth. Some forms of phenomenological research aim purely to describe rather than explain and there is also an emphasis on starting without hypotheses or preconceptions. However, many phenomenological researchers hold that the latter is simply not possible: we always approach things with preconceptions and bias, and therefore the way in which interpretations arise becomes important and should be described.

Action research

Action research aims to solve a problem. While the research is in progress, there should be changes in the organisation being studied or in the way that a particular problem is tackled. Then the research can reflect on how these changes have affected the initial problem. Initially there is a planning phase, based on understanding a problem and why it occurs. Then there is an action – the putting into effect of something predicted to improve the situation. This needs to be carefully monitored to see what effects the change has on the initial problem and to check it is not creating another problem. In a cycle there needs to be reflection before further planning and action can take place.

In reality the process in action research is much fuzzier and the steps described can and do take place concurrently. The important point is that this research is not about getting a description, a theory or simply an understanding of a phenomenon; rather, it is about enacting change and gauging the results of that change. There is also no aim to discover conclusive proof but rather an understanding that findings remain inconclusive and open to further improvement.

This approach to research can be very helpful in healthcare – for example, in evaluating public health interventions. There does not need to be a separation between researcher and research subject and the process could be undertaken by an individual or team looking at its own performance. The difference from our everyday reflective practice is that action research involves careful planning, observation and critical reflection.

Action research is often undertaken by groups with a common purpose and this is often focused on something considered a 'social good', such as improved healthcare. It is situation specific but the knowledge gained is often transferable to other situations. Action research is not necessarily qualitative but it does typically use qualitative methods such as interviews, observation and focus groups.

Pragmatic research

Pragmatic research is not a single, neat qualitative research methodology. All research methods and methodologies have limitations; pragmatic research aims to circumvent these. It also avoids getting too involved in epistemological debates by utilising the most appropriate methods at any point in the research process.

Using several methods can be very powerful because effective triangulation can occur. There can be both statistical rigour and in-depth understanding of people's lived experiences in the same research study. However, there can also be limitations, the most obvious of which is the expertise of the researchers in the research methods chosen. It is important that research methods are applied appropriately, with enough understanding of their practice, strengths and limitations to ensure adequate research findings. As with any research, it is important that there is a well-thought-out research question and the existing literature on a subject is known and understood.

QUALITATIVE RESEARCH METHODS

Q 4.9 Focus groups can provide useful data and information, but which of the following options is a limitation of focus groups?
a) They are moderated so the discussion can be kept on track.
b) They produce a limited amount of data.
c) They are simple to conduct and finding participants is easy.
d) Participants in a group tend to agree and state socially acceptable views.
e) The data produced are easily generalisable.

Q 4.10 Qualitative interviewing can be:
a) structured with responses having to be on a measurable scale
b) open to changes in the discussion topic
c) a wide variety of techniques that aim to uncover people's experiences and values
d) carefully controlled so that participants cannot change the topic
e) all of the above

Q 4.11 Which of the following is associated with the Delphi technique? Choose all of the following options that apply.
a) Seeking advice from experts
b) Seeking the views of the general population
c) Summarising the views of experts and then asking them to revise and refine these views
d) Giving expert opinion pre-eminence in qualitative research
e) Avoiding the views of the general population

There are many data collection techniques in qualitative research. Achieving better reliability and generalisability in qualitative research calls for formalised techniques that aim to reduce bias and get the best quality information and data possible. Often qualitative research aims to get as much depth as possible and this requires careful recording and reflection on the data collected. Here we discuss a few of the most common qualitative research methods.

Questionnaire design
Collecting information from people using a questionnaire is one of the most common research methodologies. It is also one of the most common methods for undertaking poor-quality research, as errors are made in questionnaire design, administration and analysis. As usual, it is important to formulate a good research question and then determine whether using a questionnaire is the correct method. If it is, then it is important to consider how the

questionnaire will obtain accurate and appropriate data and how the response rate can be maximised. Careful questionnaire design is therefore essential.

Constructing the questionnaire questions requires much thought. Are the questions going to be open ended and allow free text answers, or are they going to be closed so that the respondents have to tick a box to say yes or no, pick from a list of options or rate their response on a scale? Common scales used here are Likert scales ranging from 'strongly disagree' to 'strongly agree' or differential scales, providing a range of numbers from, for example, 1 to 10, with an extreme of response at each end. Open questions will provide a rich and varied collection of responses but may be harder to analyse. Closed questions create questionnaires that are quickly completed, with results that can be easily analysed but which may miss some important responses and hence cause frustration from respondents. It can be seen that this methodology is used in both qualitative and quantitative research.

The questions need to be short and simple and care must be taken with wording so that ambiguous words, such as 'frequently', are avoided. The questions need to be precise so that they obtain the answer required from the respondents. Questions asking for sensitive information have to be thoughtfully worded and questions asking for personal information are best placed at the end. It is a good idea to start with more general questions that are easier and more factual. It is also helpful to start with more closed questions and those obviously related to the research subject. Throughout the questionnaire, questions need to be written so that they are free of bias. Common errors are

---

Factors shown to increase response rates

- The questionnaire is clearly designed and has a simple layout
- It offers participants incentives or prizes in return for completion
- It has been thoroughly piloted and tested
- Participants are notified about the study in advance with a personalised invitation
- The aim of the study and means of completing the questionnaire are clearly explained
- A researcher is available to answer questions and collect the completed questionnaire
- If using a postal questionnaire, a stamped addressed envelope is included
- The participant feels they are a stakeholder in the study
- Questions are phrased in a way that holds the participant's attention
- The questionnaire has clear focus and purpose and is kept concise
- The questionnaire is appealing to look at, as is the researcher
- If appropriate, the questionnaire is delivered electronically

FIGURE 4.1 Factors shown to increase response rates*

---

* Adapted from Boynton PM. Administering, analysing, and reporting your questionnaire. *BMJ.* 2004; 328(7452): 1372–5.

leading questions or questions that allow the respondent to guess what the researcher wants and then answer accordingly.

The response rate is affected by many factors and a high rate is crucial if valid conclusions are to be drawn from the research (*see* Figure 4.1). How to deal with non-responders also needs to be decided.

Questionnaire design needs to account for respondents' culture, non-English-speaking groups, socially excluded groups and illiteracy rates. It needs to be decided whether the questionnaire will be self-administered, such as a postal questionnaire, or be completed by a member of the research team. Advance planning is required to decide sampling techniques and the population to be studied. All these considerations will affect the results obtained.

Many errors can be avoided by careful piloting and even more can be avoided if an already validated and published questionnaire is available to use.

Participant observation

It is possible to undertake qualitative research simply by observing particular groups of people and analysing their behaviour. This type of research aims not to be completely objective but to get subjective understanding of the research participants from their viewpoint and within their own cultural and social setting. This is *participant observation where the researcher is deeply involved in a group.*

The researcher may already be a member of the group being studied, but more likely the researcher will have to engage with the group and gain their trust. This is sometimes done secretly but ethical considerations suggest that the aims of the researcher should be open and the research participants should be fully aware of these. However, the act of observing is recognised to have an impact on the group being observed. Given this, researchers try to consider the effect their research study has on the research participants and try to minimise the impact.

This research method is time intensive and can be emotionally intensive as well. The size of the study will be limited and the group studied may not be representative of any larger population. However, insight into the group may be deep enough to understand things that may normally be covered up or secret.

The researcher must be able to engage and participate with the group being studied. This can be difficult if the group has particular attributes that the researcher does not, such as a particular age, ethnicity, gender or class. Where this is overcome the researcher can acquire a much deeper understanding of what defines the group.

Narrative-based research

Narrative analysis or inquiry uses stories, journals, letters, diaries, conversations, photos and interviews and other documentary evidence to investigate how people create narratives. People have complex lives and have complex systems for understanding their own lives. We all create narratives to make sense of the things that happen to us and other people. These narratives are often based on prevailing social mores. Narratives are formed by retrospective analysis of situations. These narratives can be drawn from a very wide range of sources, such as media, family stories and pictures, professional interventions and cultural beliefs.

The focus of narrative-based research is how knowledge and meaning is arrived at and how it is utilised. It also explores how knowledge and meaning change. This can be a very complex task and it entails the researcher looking at who constructs narratives and for whom. The researcher may also consider how those narratives differ depending on the relationships between people. For example, a patient may tell a doctor that he is worried that he has a chest infection because of shortness of breath, coughing and fevers; the same patient may downplay these symptoms to a dependent relative because he wants to avoid worrying the relative. The situation changes the narrative.

The researcher needs to consider how to gather narratives and explore them but also how to present them. Sometimes fiction is very powerful, not because of the actual narrative but because of how it chimes with the reader. This is also true of narrative research reports. They are open to further interpretation and narrative forming. This requires the researcher to be open about how he or she has uncovered the narratives and how he or she has attributed meaning.

There are debates about the authenticity of narrative research reports – can a researcher claim to know, understand and have the authority to present other people's narratives? The narrative the researcher presents has to be recognised as the narrative of the researcher as much as, if not more than, the narrative of the research subject.

Interviews

Interviewing is of course not unique to qualitative data collection – it is extensively used in large data collection surveys. Interviews can take many different forms but there is a distinction between structured and unstructured interviews. *Structured interviews aim to deliver data that are consistent and do not vary depending on the interviewer,* as many interviewers may be employed to collect large data sets. Structured interviews can provide data that are comparable between areas and over time when well designed and appropriately conducted. The disadvantage of structured interviews is that they can mask individual variety and they do not target a depth of understanding.

Unstructured interviews allow for much more freedom in the kind of data collected. The interviewer can follow up on anything the interviewee says and consider it in more depth. This is often useful when researchers are trying to get the perspectives of a particular group of people and want to understand their experiences, motivations or decision-making processes in detail.

Semi-structured interviews are a halfway point whereby there is a structure and a set of questions that are used to open the interview and used at points within it but the interviewer still has freedom to follow up on interesting comments by the interviewee. The idea is to gain as much depth of understanding as possible from the interview. These techniques are useful to elucidate on findings from quantitative questionnaires. They are also useful when there is a range of subjects the researchers are interested in and more detailed data are required.

Focus groups

Sometimes *interviews are held with several people rather than an individual*. These can provide a very different dynamic, where the researcher wants the participants to debate among themselves. This is often described as a focus group. There are different ways of convening a focus group. People with a particular interest or expertise in an area may be invited to participate, but often the people invited represent a broad cross-section of the population. The researcher will facilitate discussion and steer it when necessary. There needs to be guidance for both group participants and facilitators in order to enable useful information to be recorded and to avoid digression.

One of the downsides to focus groups is that you need an appropriate mix of people for the questions being asked. If the group has no interest in the questions or fails to engage with them, the data will not be very helpful. Also, if there are dominant and submissive personalities in the group, then certain viewpoints may be focused on, to the detriment of other possibly more thoughtful or valid perspectives. Another disadvantage is that the participants may not reflect the broader population of interest and so may give potentially misleading results.

Delphi technique

The Delphi technique comes from forecasting techniques that aim to get several experts in a field to predict events. After an initial round in which a panel of experts answer a questionnaire, the summary of the results from all the experts is fed back and each one is asked to refine his or her views. This may occur several times. The idea is to break down a complex problem to enable a consensus to be reached, particularly where there are no data and there are time pressures.

The researcher does not need to be an expert in the field but he or she does need to be able to summarise the important points and feed this back effectively. Often the experts remain anonymous, to encourage them to give their honest opinion. They are also given the chance to modify their views based on knowing what other experts have suggested. The process is stopped at a predetermined point, which may be a predetermined number of rounds or when a close enough consensus is reached.

There are several modifications to the Delphi technique, including methods that can be used in focus groups and meetings; its use has also been extended into policymaking. The disadvantage of this technique is that experts are not always correct and the consensus opinion may not adequately reflect the most accurate opinions in the group.

QUALITATIVE DATA ANALYSIS

Qualitative research can lead to a great diversity of data and information. This presents challenges in terms of what to do with the data collected. There are numerous ways of dealing with the collected data and the ways a researcher chooses are based on the researcher's epistemological standpoint, his or her need for generalisable results, and practical issues such as time and money.

Analysing qualitative data sets can lead to insights that were not obvious during the course of the data collection. Putting together themes from different data collection techniques can reinforce or dispute ideas or theories about the research subjects.

Once the data have been collected, there is often some form of coding – assigning data to a theme in order to see links with other pieces of data. The themes may arise from the theoretical background of the research or they may arise from the actual data. Themes could include significant phrases used by members of a group or expressed preferences. Once the data have been coded, they can be analysed and described. This may lead to further data collection or questions that require further research.

Sometimes there is no formal method of data analysis. Researchers may pick up on specific aspects of their research and explore that in conjunction with hypotheses and theories framed via a literature review. They may write a narrative account of the research. There may even be fictional accounts of the research that aim to show an understanding of several of the research participants. This can be more emotive than an academic paper.

The diversity of data analysis techniques means that qualitative research may not give a reader the information that he or she desires. This can be a strength if it exposes readers to ideas that they may not have previously considered. However, it can be frustrating for a healthcare worker who simply wants to know how best to tackle the problems faced by his or her patients. This is why quantitative research results can be very helpful in conjunction with qualitative research results. Mixed research can strengthen the comprehension of a particular patient experience.

In the next chapter we look at quantitative research techniques.

CHAPTER 5

Quantitative methods

INTRODUCTION

Quantitative methods entail the use of research methods that lead to numerical out-comes. These outcomes can then be analysed with statistical methods to provide information about diagnostic tests, treatments and interventions, and, potentially, how selected attributes affect people's health. At their most simple, they take two variables and try to work out whether they are related and if so by how much. An obvious example in medicine would be trying to ascertain how useful a drug is for treating a particular condition.

In order to have good, reliable information we need good study designs with appropriate outcome measures. In this chapter we look at study designs and the data that studies provide. For the AKT you need to have a grasp of the different types of study design, their advantages and disadvantages and also how to interpret common outcome measures such as relative risk and odds ratios.

Q 5.1 Match the type of study (left) with the most appropriate definition (right).

a) Randomised controlled trial	1) Prospective study looking at how people are affected by exposure to risk factors
b) Meta-analysis	2) Study participants are randomly allocated to one or more interventions
c) Cohort study	3) A summary of several studies
d) Expert opinion	4) Subjects with a particular disease are studied to determine exposure to a predicted cause
e) Case-control study	5) The experience and considered opinion of people working in a particular field

Q 5.2 Put the following items in the order in which they appear in the hierarchy of evidence, starting with the highest level of evidence.

a) Cohort studies
b) Case series and case reports
c) Randomised controlled trials
d) Case-control studies
e) Systematic reviews and meta-analyses
f) Expert opinion

THE HIERARCHY OF EVIDENCE

The 'hierarchy of evidence' (shown in Figure 5.1) is a scheme that ranks types of evidence and how much importance we can ascribe to the results of a well-conducted study of each type. It is commonly used when evaluating evidence for the production of guidance. The hierarchy of evidence is based solely on the type of data or information provided by the different levels in the hierarchy, but this is idealised. The hierarchy on its own does not determine how useful an individual study may be. You need to understand the context of a study in order to evaluate it. Just because you are reading a systematic review containing meta-analyses does not mean that the answers will be either authoritative or applicable to questions that you have. It is worth repeating that understanding the context of evidence is absolutely vital in knowing what it tells us.

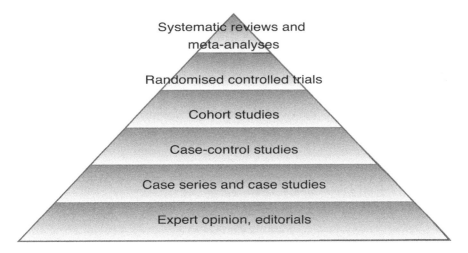

FIGURE 5.1 One version of the hierarchy of evidence: this shows the most robust evidence at the top of the pyramid

Randomised controlled trials (RCTs) are seen as the gold standard for medical trials. If they are well designed, appropriately conducted and accurately reported, they give some of the most useful and reliable information available to clinicians. It is rare that a single RCT will give a complete and authoritative answer to a clinical question. Therefore, we need ways of combining the results of RCTs. This can be provided by meta-analyses or systematic reviews. These sit at the top of the hierarchy of evidence, because they synthesise data and findings from several studies to provide an overview of the state of evidence regarding a particular subject. Perhaps the best-known examples are those that the Cochrane Collaboration provides (if you have not used the Cochrane Library already, then take a look at the reviews that it has conducted, as many are directly applicable to general practice).*

It is not always appropriate to use an RCT to answer a clinical question. If, for example, you want to know more about the prognosis of patients following a stroke, you may choose to perform a longitudinal study following a group of patients (a cohort study) or even a descriptive study of an individual patient (a case report).

If you wanted to know the accuracy of a diagnostic test for a rare disease, a cross-sectional or possibly a cohort study may be most useful. So do not be fooled into thinking that studies higher up the hierarchy of evidence are intrinsically better than those that are lower.

Remember that the questions that arise in day-to-day clinical practice *may* be best answered by qualitative research (*see* Chapter 4), which is not normally included in the hierarchy of evidence. As GPs we often find that understanding the experience of patients is more helpful than knowing which is the most efficacious drug for a particular condition. For example, a patient who comes to see you following the death of a family member will not need you to have a firm grasp of guidelines for treating depression and comparative selective serotonin reuptake inhibitor efficacy, but the patient *will* need you to be able to listen and possibly provide a little insight into grieving processes.

Let us take a look at each of the levels of the hierarchy of evidence in turn, starting with the top of the pyramid and working down. This is not a comprehensive list of study design; indeed, some studies do not easily fit into any particular category. For the AKT you should have an understanding of how each type of study is conducted, its strengths and weaknesses and how to interpret the outcomes.

---

* www.cochrane.org

SYSTEMATIC REVIEWS AND META-ANALYSIS

Q 5.3   What is the difference between a systematic review and meta-analysis? Choose the most appropriate single answer from the following options.
a) A systematic review combines results of trials into a single mathematical model; a meta-analysis does not.
b) A meta-analysis is based on every trial on a particular subject, whereas a systematic review has more tightly defined criteria.
c) A meta-analysis shows data in a graphical format, whereas a systematic review uses narrative.
d) A systematic review uses defined criteria to answer a defined question; a meta-analysis is a quantitative combination of results from several studies.
e) A systematic review has a tightly focused research question; it uses defined criteria to answer that question. A meta-analysis uses weighted averages of all the studies on a particular subject.

Q 5.4   Look at the following diagram. What is this type of graph called?

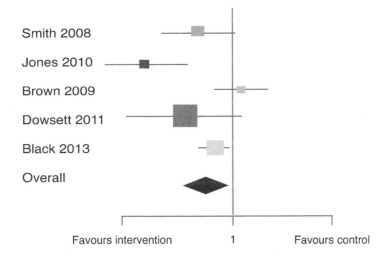

a) A funnel plot
b) A forest plot
c) A leaf-and-branch plot
d) Relative risk summary
e) A Tudor Jones plot

Q 5.5 Looking at the diagram in Question 5.4, match each of the following definitions (below left) to the following descriptions (below right). Each answer is used only once

a) This sign represents pooled data from all trials shown

b) This represents the 95% confidence interval of each study

c) This is the line of no effect and is associated with a relative risk or odds ratio of 1

d) This often correlates to the size of each trial

e) This represents the effect of the intervention found in each study

1) The square in the middle of each line

2) Size of the square on each horizontal line

3) Width of each horizontal line

4) Solid vertical line

5) Diamond below all horizontal lines

The idea behind systematic reviews is that a research question can be answered in a way that limits bias to ensure more reliable and accurate conclusions. The advantages of systematic reviews are summarised in Figure 5.2. Systematic reviews are secondary research; this means that they use results from other studies and collate them. Primary studies are those that actually collect original data.

Advantages of systematic reviews

- Bias is limited through the use of explicit criteria and methods.
- A clearly focused question is stated, allowing its relevance to your practice to be assessed.
- Because methods are explicitly reported the review can be easily repeated and therefore updated as new evidence becomes available.
- Doctors and others needing accurate information can easily find the most robust conclusions about clinically focused questions.
- Studies are compared to identify the extent of generalisability and validity of their results.
- If heterogeneity (inconsistency or difference) between studies is identified, the reasons for this may be identified and therefore new research questions and hypotheses may be generated.
- Good-quality, up-to-date systematic reviews may decrease the time that research findings take to be put into clinical practice.

FIGURE 5.2 A summary of the advantages of systematic reviews

A systematic review is a look at a particular subject or question, which means searching for *all* the relevant studies with an explicit search strategy and then evaluating the studies against predetermined criteria. This means searching systematically, looking for both published and unpublished studies, trying to find every study that may be relevant. Then the studies need to be assessed for relevance to the systematic review topic, and the studies need to be assessed for quality. There are established guidelines that set out how to assess the quality of a study, but briefly it means looking to see whether appropriate methods were used, whether the reported outcomes are appropriate and ensuring that there is as little bias as possible in a study. Once the studies have been assessed, some will be rejected because of inadequate quality or not being directly relevant to the review question. Then the results can be combined in a meta-analysis.

A meta-analysis is the combining of the selected study results by mathematical means. Combining the results of two or more studies can give more conclusive answers. This is because effectively the number of people studied is increased, reducing the confidence interval of the results (*see* Chapter 3). Each of the selected studies can be given a weighting in the analysis based on how reliable and useful that study has been found to be. This is often related to the number of study participants. A common way of representing results of meta-analyses is a forest plot. This is a graphical representation of trial results (as seen in Question 5.4), showing the size or weighting of the study, the confidence interval for the results of each trial and an overall result combining the results of all the selected trials.

The studies included in the meta-analysis are listed down the left side of the graph. Be aware that occasionally the layout may be turned on its side – this fits with the convention of having the independent variables on the y-axis but it is rarely used by medical researchers. The blob (hence blobbogram – another name for a forest plot), or square, on the horizontal line is centred on the point estimate (the actual value of the relative risk (RR) or odds ratio (OR), or other chosen measurement) of the effect of the studied interventions. The width of the horizontal line represents the 95% confidence interval of the relative risk or odds ratio estimate. This is often shown numerically down the right-hand side of the graph. Remember that any of the horizontal lines that cross the solid vertical line do not have a statistically significant effect. *The solid vertical line is the line of no effect* – if it is relative risk, odds ratios or hazard ratios that are plotted, this will have a value of 1.

The overall summary, or more accurately the pooled result, of the trials based on the statistical combination of all the studies is shown by the diamond at the bottom of the figure just above the x-axis. The tips of the diamond represent the confidence interval of the overall result; if one of these touches or crosses the solid vertical line it means that there is no statistically significant difference between the study outcomes. Remember that this needs to be interpreted with an understanding not only of the question that the meta-analysis was trying to answer but also of the quality and size of the studies included in the meta-analysis. If all the studies are relatively small it is possible that the result is not statistically significant, because larger studies are needed to show relatively small differences in outcomes. As with all statistical results, you need to know what has been measured and why.

Disadvantages of meta-analyses

- There may be significant publication bias, which will affect the overall result. Negative results are less often reported and this will make a meta-analysis have a more positive outcome.

- There may be other bias in the selected studies – for example, incomplete reporting of results.

- The context of each of the primary studies may not be directly comparable; for example, the study populations may be very different in age and social class, they may live in very different locations, they may have very different levels of co-morbidity and they may be studied over very different time frames.

- The designs of the primary studies may mean combining results is not appropriate.

- Not all meta-analyses are free of bias with explicit methods and careful results.

FIGURE 5.3 A brief summary of disadvantages of systematic reviews

Q 5.6 Another type of graph that is sometimes seen in systematic reviews and meta-analyses is provided here. What does this graph show?

19 studies comparing two drugs for effectiveness in treating glaucoma

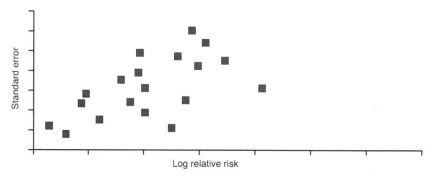

Treatment effect against standard error of the study

a) That there is likely to be publication bias
b) That there is no statistically significant correlation between these variables
c) That there is a statistically significant correlation between these variables
d) That the topic needs further research
e) That it is unlikely that there is publication bias in these results

This is a funnel plot, so called because the graph should have a funnel shape. These are useful in systematic reviews and meta-analyses to look for, among other things, evidence that not all the available data have been published (this is called **publication bias**[*]). It tends to be negative studies that do not get published. However, these studies are not irrelevant and still provide useful information; if you want to know how good an intervention is, you need to know about possible side effects and see evidence of ineffectiveness.

A funnel plot is based on the assumption that larger studies will be more powerful and precise and therefore be nearer the true value than smaller studies, which should be spread on both sides of that value. The intervention effect (in the funnel plot shown in Q5.6, this is plotted as log relative risk on the x-axis) estimates are plotted against a measure of the studies' precision or size (in the funnel plot shown, this is plotted on the y-axis as standard error). If the scatter plot of trials is asymmetrical around the true value, this suggests that not all the studies in the field have been published. The graph in Question 5.6 is asymmetrical, as there are fewer studies to the right side of the graph. However, be aware that asymmetry can be due to systematic differences between smaller and larger studies or use of inappropriate measures or even higher dropout rates in some studies.

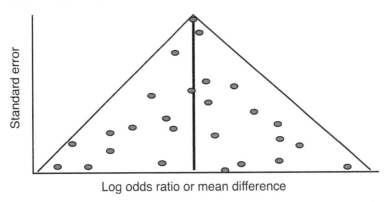

FIGURE 5.4 A symmetrical funnel plot, suggesting no publication bias

Figure 5.4 is an example of a funnel plot with good symmetry, suggesting no publication bias. The solid lines showing the funnel shape are the boundaries within which 95% of studies would be expected to fall if there is no bias or heterogeneity. Heterogeneity refers to differences in study results that are not attributable to chance alone. For example, variability in the participants,

---

* See Egger M, Davey Smith G, Schneider M, *et al.* Bias in meta-analysis detected by a simple, graphical test. *BMJ.* 1997; **315**(7109): 629–34. See also Sterne JA, Sutton AJ, Ioannidis JP, *et al.* Recommendations for examining and interpreting funnel plot asymmetry in meta-analyses of randomised controlled trials. *BMJ.* 2011; **343**: d4002.

interventions, study designs and risk of bias will all result in variability in the intervention effects seen. *Heterogeneity is a measure of how different studies are. Homogeneity is a measure of how similar studies are.*

Q 5.7 A systematic review and meta-analysis is performed looking at the effects of intensive blood pressure lowering (i.e. reducing blood pressure to below 140/90) on cardiovascular and renal outcomes. The review found that more intensive blood pressure-lowering interventions reduced the risk of major cardiovascular events by 11% (RR 0.89, 95% confidence interval 0.79–0.99, p = 0.036) compared to less intensive interventions.* Which of the following statements are true?

a) Patients with higher blood pressure were more likely to have a cardiovascular event.

b) Lowering blood pressure meant patients were less likely to have a cardiovascular event.

c) Intensively lowering blood pressure leads to less frequent major cardiovascular events.

d) Because the upper limit of the confidence interval is 0.99, there may not be any benefit in intensive blood pressure-lowering regimens.

e) None of the above are true.

Q 5.8 The same trial produced the following forest plot.

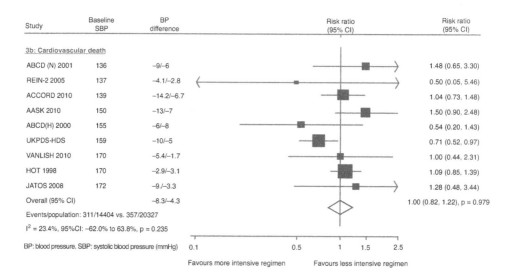

BP: blood pressure, SBP: systolic blood pressure (mmHg)

---

* Lv J, Neal B, Ehteshami P, *et al.* Effects of intensive blood pressure lowering on cardiovascular and renal outcomes: a systematic review and meta-analysis. *PLoS Med.* 2012; 9(8): e1001293.

Q 5.9   Which of the trials has a statistically significant outcome? Write your answer in the box.

```
                                                        
```

Q 5.10 Is the overall result of the meta-analysis statistically significant?
Yes ☐   No ☐

Q 5.11 Were cardiovascular deaths reduced by intensive blood pressure-lowering regimens?
Yes ☐   No ☐

Q 5.12 Which study was given the greatest weighting in the meta-analysis?
a) REIN-2 2005
b) VANLISH 2010
c) ABCD (N) 2001
d) JATOS 2008
e) HOT 1998

The answer to Question 5.7 is C – this is a question about accurate interpretation of results. It may well be that both A and B are also true but we cannot know this from the results presented here. Statements A and B both include 'cardiovascular events', not **major** cardiovascular events, and therefore would include all cardiovascular events. It is possible that there was no significant difference in the number of all cardiovascular events between normal and intensive blood pressure-lowering regimens. We only know that **major** cardiovascular events were found to be less likely with intensive antihypertensive regimens. Note also that this can only be considered to be true over the time frame of the study. Longer-term follow-up may well produce different results. The answer D does not make sense because the confidence interval does not encompass 1; therefore there is a statistically significant effect.

The forest plot shows trials that included cardiovascular death as an outcome from intensive and less intensive blood pressure-lowering regimens. Looking at the forest plot, the only trial with a confidence interval that does not cross the line of no effect is the UKPDS-HDS trial. This is therefore the only statistically significant trial included in the meta-analysis.

The overall result shows the diamond sitting over the line of no effect; therefore, there is no statistically significant result from combining the results of all the trials. This demonstrates how meta-analyses can show that trials that have produced a statistically significant result are not always correct. Remember that where a confidence interval of 95% is used in trials it is probable that one in 20 trials will find a statistically significant result even when there is no actual relationship between the variables being studied.

The overall conclusion from this part of the meta-analysis is that there is no reduction in cardiovascular deaths from an intensive blood pressure-reducing regimen. Reading the systematic review that it is based on will show that what is considered an intensive regimen varies greatly by paper. This reiterates how important it is to read the meta-analysis methods and discussion before drawing firm conclusions of your own.

The HOT trial published in 1998 was given the greatest weighting in this meta-analysis. You can tell this because the square representing it is the largest of the options given in the question. The reasons that it was given the greatest weighting include the size of the study and the methods used in that study.

RANDOMISED CONTROLLED TRIALS

As already mentioned, RCTs are considered the gold standard of research studies. A well-conducted RCT with an appropriate research objective should provide useful information with the minimum of bias. This is especially helpful when looking at the effects of drugs and therapeutic interventions. Making sure that both research participants and researchers are unaware of which intervention or placebo is being given to each participant is the best way of ensuring there is as little bias as possible in a study. *This is called double-blinding, because both researchers and participants are blinded to who is receiving which intervention or placebo.*

The most useful RCTs are those that compare an intervention and the existing gold standard treatment. These give outcomes that can be directly translated into practice. However, it has to be remembered that there are financial constraints on healthcare systems and therefore cost needs to be considered when deciding whether an intervention is worth using or not. The National Institute for Health and Care Excellence clinical guidance always has an economic evaluation and comparison of possible interventions. There is a section on economic analysis in Chapter 6.

Advantages of RCTs include that bias should be minimised (remember that you will need to read the methods section of a paper to know how good the study is and whether bias has been effectively eliminated). They should also deliver good-quality, useful data, which enables more sophisticated analysis.

If there is effective blinding alongside effective randomisation, there should be an equal distribution of all the attributes of the research participants that could affect the results.

The biggest disadvantages of RCTs are that they are very costly to do effectively, there is a need to have a large number of research participants in order to make the results more useful and the need for blinding makes them more difficult to do. There can also be ethical problems – for example, how do you do RCTs with effective blinding when looking at surgical interventions? Is it appropriate to use sham operations on patients?

Advantages	Disadvantages
• Unbiased distribution of confounders	• Expensive
• Blinding of participants and researchers	• Time-consuming
• More powerful statistical analysis possible	• There can be ethical problems

FIGURE 5.5 A brief summary of the advantages and disadvantages of randomised controlled trials

A type of modified RCT is a crossover trial, which gives a group of participants an intervention and then after an appropriate time period gives them another intervention. This can be cheaper to do than an RCT. It can also be helpful where it is thought unethical to not give a particular treatment to all the study participants. The obvious disadvantages are that although participants are their own controls, there can be effects that are based on the order in which participants are given interventions and the effect of one intervention may not have disappeared fully before the next intervention is given. This type of study cannot be used where the effects of an intervention are long-lasting or permanent. The washout period is the time allowed for effects of an intervention to have disappeared before starting another treatment. To avoid bias arising from the order in which treatments are given, these studies can split participants into two groups: one of the groups has the interventions in the order A then B; the other group has the interventions in the order B then A.

Absolute and relative risk

Q 5.13 Match the following equations (right) with the correct test (left).

Test	Equation
a) Relative risk increase or reduction	CER − EER
b) Number needed to treat or harm	$\dfrac{(a/c)}{(b/d)}$
c) Odds ratio	$\dfrac{(\text{CER} - \text{EER})}{\text{CER}}$
d) Absolute risk increase or reduction	$\dfrac{1}{(\text{CER} - \text{EER})}$
e) Relative risk	$\dfrac{\text{EER}}{\text{CER}}$

Note: CER means control event rate and EER means experimental event rate.

Answers are in the text.

RCTs normally use the absolute or relative risk reduction or increase to evaluate interventions. Expect a question on relative or absolute risk in the AKT exam. In this context, risk does not mean a hazard or danger: it can be understood to be synonymous to the probability of a particular event occurring. Obviously this is often a positive thing – for example, the reduction in the chance of cardiovascular events in people taking metformin for diabetes. The difference between absolute and relative is that relative measurements are a comparison with something other than zero; in the case of relative risk, this is a **comparison** of risk in the experimental group to risk in a control group.

Absolute risk (AR) is the chance (or actual risk) of developing a condition, with zero meaning there is no risk. In the context of an RCT, *absolute risk reduction or increase (ARR or ARI) is the **difference** in risk in those subjected to the experimental intervention.* The control group is used to determine the baseline risk when the intervention is not used.

The control event rate (CER) is a measure of how often the event of interest occurs in the control group. The experimental event rate (EER) is how often that event occurs in the group given the intervention being studied. For example, the chance of cardiovascular death in a control group (study participants in this group may be treated with what is considered to be the normal best treatment available) may be compared with the chance of cardiovascular death in a group taking high-dose statins.

Absolute risk reduction or increase

$$CER - EER$$

Note that with this equation, if the change in absolute risk is greater than zero then this is a risk reduction, because in the experimental group there is a lower rate of the condition of interest than in the control group. If the change in absolute risk is less than zero then this is a risk increase; this means that the event rate in the experimental group is bigger than the event rate in the control group.

Relative risk reduction or increase is the **ratio** *of the probability of an outcome in the experimental group compared with the probability of the same outcome in the control, or comparison, group.* Relative risk does not tell you what the actual risk is; it only tells us the risk in comparison with another group. Relative risk reduction or increase often appears to give much bigger changes in risk than the absolute risk reduction or increase, and for this reason it is important to always know the absolute risk as well.

For example, an RCT shows that taking a beta blocker as secondary prevention alongside an ACE inhibitor (ACE-I) reduces all-cause mortality by 2% per year (the absolute risk reduction) compared with taking an ACE-I alone. If the risk of dying per annum for people taking only an ACE-I is 6% per year (the CER) this is reduced to 4% (the EER) in the group taking both a beta blocker and an ACE-I, giving a relative risk reduction of a third, or 33%. The absolute risk reduction is 6% minus 4% = 2% but the relative risk is reduced by 33%. The latter figure is obviously much more attention grabbing. If you were told that prescribing a drug caused a 33% reduction in mortality, you would immediately be more impressed than if you were told that it caused a 2% reduction in mortality.

When presented with a figure from a study, always work out if it is a relative or absolute risk reduction. If the figure is relative risk reduction, you then need to know the baseline figures – that is, what is the absolute risk of a particular event before taking the intervention.

You need to know how to calculate relative risk reduction or increase. If you remember that relative risk reduction or increase is a ratio, it will be easier to remember how to calculate it. Ratios are where one number is divided by another. To find the relative risk reduction or increase you have to divide the absolute risk reduction or increase by the control event rate.

Relative risk reduction or increase

$$\frac{CER - EER}{CER}$$

Remember for absolute risk reduction or increase, a result greater than 0 is a risk reduction and a result less than 0 is a risk increase. For relative risk (and also any other ratios such as the odds ratio) a value of 1 signifies no difference between the groups being studied (because 1 will be the result if you divide a number by itself). This is why if a relative risk or odds ratio result has a confidence interval that crosses the value 1, it has to be concluded that no significant effect has been found. Relative risk is looked at again in the section on cohort studies later in this chapter.

Hazard ratio

A hazard ratio is similar to relative risk ratios but it takes into account the timing of events. This is useful particularly in survival analysis; where once a patient has reached the end point of a study (for example, death or cure) they no longer need to be included in the analysis. A hazard is the rate at which events happen. These events do not have to be hazardous in the general meaning of the term; they can include positive events.

A hazard ratio compares the hazard of events in the treatment arm of a trial with the hazard of the events occurring in the control arm. The calculation for the hazard ratio involves hazard rates over the entire duration of a study and can be derived from a Kaplan–Meier curve (*see* Chapter 6). It is often used in RCTs but can also be used in survival analysis. A hazard ratio of 1 corresponds to the relative probability in the two groups being equal over time; a hazard ratio above 1 signifies a raised hazard for the treatment group; a hazard ratio below 1 a decreased hazard for the treatment group; a hazard ratio of 0.5 means that half as many patients in the active group have an event compared with the control group.

We will not give a formula for hazard ratios, as there are several of these and they are more complicated than you would be expected to know for the AKT. However, it is useful to understand hazard ratios for when looking at journal articles and trial reports.

The number needed to treat and number needed to harm

The number needed to treat (NNT) (or number needed to harm, NNH) is found from the absolute risk reduction or increase. It is simply the inverse of the absolute risk reduction (1/ARR); which shows how many people would have to be treated to prevent (or cause) one outcome of interest. This is a useful way of assessing the effectiveness of an intervention. For example, in patients who have had a myocardial infarction, the number needed to treat with a beta blocker to prevent one death in the year following their myocardial infarction is

25 according to the Norwegian Multicenter Study on Timolol after Myocardial Infarction.[*] Note that other studies have found different NNTs.

Note that in order to have an accurate and useful statistic, you need to specify what your outcome of interest is (in this case, all-cause mortality), the intervention that is being considered (secondary prevention with beta blockers) and over what time frame (for example, over 1 year). (The NNT over more than 1 year would be lower because there is more time for effects to be seen.)

Number needed to treat or harm

$$\frac{1}{CER - EER}$$

It is very likely that there will be a question in the AKT paper that requires you to remember one of the formulas outlined so far in this chapter. Try to commit them to memory for the AKT.

Q 5.14 The results from a study are shown in the following table. How many study participants were there? Write your answer in the box below the table.

	Control group	Experimental group	Total
Events	20	10	30
Non-events	80	90	170
Total number of participants	100	100	200

Q 5.15 What is the absolute risk reduction?
a) 5%
b) 10%
c) 20%
d) 80%
e) 90%

* Pedersen TR. The Norwegian multicentre study on Timolol after myocardial infarction – design, management and results on mortality. *Acta Medica Scandinavica*. 1981; **210**(S651): 235–41.

Q **5.16** What is the relative risk reduction?
  a) 5%
  b) 10%
  c) 50%
  d) 75%
  e) 80%

Q **5.17** What is the number needed to treat?
  a) 1
  b) 2
  c) 10
  d) 20
  e) 50

The number of study participants is very easy to calculate: 200. This is adding together the total number of study participants in both the control and the experimental arms of the study. The control event rate (CER) is 0.2 (20/100 = 20%) and the experimental event rate (EER) is 0.1 (10/100 = 10%).

  Therefore, the absolute risk reduction is:

$$\text{CER} - \text{EER} = 0.2 - 0.1 = 0.1 = 10\%$$

The relative risk reduction is:

$$\frac{\text{CER} - \text{EER}}{\text{CER}} = \frac{0.2 - 0.1}{0.2} = \frac{0.1}{0.2} = 0.5 \;\; = 50\%$$

The number needed to treat is:

$$= \frac{1}{\text{CER} - \text{EER}} = \frac{1}{0.2 - 0.1} = \frac{1}{0.1} = 10$$

These are very simple results so that you get used to plugging the numbers into the equations. Obviously, expect harder mathematics in exam questions, but you should be able to work out the correct answer using mental arithmetic, pen and paper, or it may be quicker to work out an approximate answer using simpler numbers. For example, if there are 40 events in a control group of 426 (9.3%), this is close enough to a rate of 10%; you could use this figure to give reasonable estimates of absolute risk reduction (ARR), relative risk reduction (RRR) and number needed to treat (NNT), and probably be able to do the maths much more quickly.

  Practise questions as much as possible until you are certain you know the formulas. When doing one of these mathematical questions, try to check that the answer you arrive at makes sense in the context of what you are told in the question. Again doing many of these types of question will make this much easier – you will remember that the inverse of 40% is 2.5, for example, and this will make working out approximate NNTs far easier. You also need to know the formulas for working out relative risk and odds ratios. These will be covered in the next couple of sections.

COHORT STUDIES

A cohort study takes a group of people and sees what happens to them over time; this is known as a longitudinal study. This type of study is normally used to try to see whether suspected risk factors actually have an impact on people's health and if so, what size of impact they have. There are usually several variables that the researchers are interested in.

A cohort is a group of people who have a characteristic in common; this may be that they are of a similar age, they live in the same area, they have been treated with a particular drug or procedure or they are from a similar socio-economic or ethnic group. There may or may not be a comparison group. Sometimes there will be a group who have not had the particular exposure that the researchers are interested in – for example, smokers and non-smokers.*

Subgroups within the cohort may be compared with each other – for example, smokers and non-smokers within the cohort of people who work in a particular section of the chemical industry. Because study participants are not randomly given treatments or blinded, there is a risk that confounding variables exist – that is, there may appear to be a correlation between factors that is actually spurious because a third variable has not been taken into account.

These studies are normally 'prospective' – that is, they are looking forward in time. This avoids inaccurate recall leading to recall bias (*see* Chapter 3). Retrospective cohort studies are possible by looking at the medical records of a cohort of people to find information about variables the researchers are interested in.

Like all studies, the research design needs to be carefully considered to ascertain whether there is any bias present. For example, if a cohort study only contacts participants infrequently and then asks them what has happened in the intervening period, there will be significant recall bias in the results. One of the most famous cohort studies is the Framingham Heart Study, which has

---

* The British Doctors Study by Richard Doll and Austin Bradford Hill (later joined by Richard Peto) provided compelling evidence that smoking was harmful. They recruited a cohort of doctors in 1951 by writing to all registered doctors in the UK. See Doll R, Hill A. The mortality of doctors in relation to their smoking habits [Reprinted from *Br Med J*. 1954; 1(4877): 1451–5]. *BMJ*. 2004; **328**(7455): 1529–33.

given us a lot of information on the factors that contribute to heart disease. The results from this study can be used in general practice in an algorithm that provides an estimate of a patient's risk of having a cardiovascular event over a specified period of time.

The advantages and disadvantages of cohort studies are summed up in Figure 5.6.

Advantages	Disadvantages
• Often cheaper and easier than an RCT	• Not randomised or blinded, need large cohorts
• Can study causal relationships and determine the timing of exposure and consequence.	• Determining causality often requires further studies
• Can determine (rare) risk factors for diseases	• Not very useful for rare diseases
• Able to measure incidence	• Time-consuming to produce useful data
• Multiple outcomes can be studied	• Potential for confounding
• Exposure suspicion bias can be avoided (more of a problem in case-control studies)	• Can be subject to attrition – study participants withdrawing.

FIGURE 5.6 Brief summary of the advantages and disadvantages of cohort studies

Relative risk

The **normal** outcome measure from a cohort study is relative risk – for example, what is the risk of a cardiovascular event for someone who smokes **relative** to the risk of a cardiovascular event for someone who does not smoke. Remember from the section on relative risk reduction or increase in the RCT section that relative risk is a ratio and therefore we are dividing event rates. The probability of an event occurring in the exposed group is divided by the probability of the event happening in the non-exposed group to find relative risk.

As we have seen, *relative risk is the ratio of the probability of an outcome in one group compared with the probability of the same outcome in a comparison group.* One group needs to be exposed to a risk factor or treatment that the other group is not exposed to. A relative risk of 1 signifies that there is no measured difference between the groups studied.

Relative risk

$$\frac{\text{exposure event rate}}{\text{CER}}$$

Note that this is a little different but related to the formula for the relative risk reduction or increase we looked at in the RCT section. Expressed as a formula, the relationship between relative risk (RR) and the relative risk reduction (RRR) is RRR = 1 − RR. For example if the relative risk of having a disease is 0.8 (that is, 80%) in people taking a certain drug compared with a control group (which would have the value 1 because the RR is comparing the risk of disease in one group to that in the control group) then the relative risk reduction between the groups is 1 − 0.8 = 0.2 (or a 20% relative risk reduction).

Q 5.18 A study followed a cohort of nurses for 10 years with the following results. What is the relative risk of having lung cancer for a nurse who smokes in this study?

Risk factor	Lung cancer status	
	Lung cancer present	No lung cancer
Smoker	25	75
Non-smoker	1	99

    a) 2.5
    b) 5
    c) 25
    d) 50
    e) 100

The numbers used here are deliberately simple. It is clear that 25% of the smokers developed lung cancer (25 out of a total of 100), whereas 1% of the non-smokers developed lung cancer (1 out of 100).
    Therefore, the equation for relative risk is:

$$\frac{\text{exposure event rate}}{\text{CER}} = \frac{25/100}{1/100} = \frac{0.25}{0.01} = 25$$

That is, there is a 25 times greater chance of developing lung cancer in smokers than in non-smokers in this hypothetical study.

CASE-CONTROL STUDIES

This type of study compares people with a condition to those who do not have it. This is in order to evaluate potential causes of the condition or the risk factors that contribute to the way in which it develops. These studies are retro-spective and so rely heavily on people recalling past events relatively accurately. However, these studies are useful where the condition being studied is rare and a cohort study would be unlikely to result in having enough people with the condition to enable any meaningful analysis around the condition in question.

'Condition' does not necessarily mean illness or disease: it could be something that is beneficial to people, such as people who have immunity to particular infectious diseases. Also remember that these studies can be subject to a lot of confounding where correlations may be due to hidden or unstudied factors (spurious correlation, *see* Chapter 3). For example, a study may find that people who develop pancreatic cancer are more likely to be exposed to statins but it may also be true that people on statins are more likely to have higher risks of pancreatic cancer because of lifestyle factors and other diseases – smoking, obesity and diabetes, for example.[*]

A case-control study can be exploratory – a 'fishing expedition' – where cases and controls are selected and a variety of factors are examined to determine if they are related to the outcome. This can be valuable in identifying potential risk factors that can then be studied in greater detail, particularly when there is an urgent need for information, such as during epidemics, when the source of the outbreak is useful to know.

However, analytic case-control studies are more robust and are designed to test existing hypotheses of which factors influence a particular outcome. Study participants are recruited based on their already-known outcome status (cases and controls) and then the hypothesis tested by looking for exposure to the causative factor. It is necessary to carefully define what constitutes a case and a non-case and use the same techniques to look for exposure in all participants. It is important that controls come from a similar population to the cases and they should be subject to the same exclusions and restrictions placed on cases. It is obvious that there will be confounding and bias present in poorly designed case-control studies, but also that carefully designed case-control studies can give us valuable information. The advantages and disadvantages are summarised in Figure 5.7.

---

[*] It has been suggested that statins are an aetiological agent for pancreatic cancer, based on an increased incidence of gastrointestinal cancers in people with low cholesterol levels reported in several epidemiological studies from the 1970s and 1980s. However, several studies have found no evidence of a link; in fact it is now thought that statins may have a protective effect. See, for example, Bradley MC, Hughes CM, Cantwell MM, *et al.* Statins and pancreatic cancer risk: a nested case-control study. *Cancer Causes Control.* 2010; 21(12): 2093–100.

Advantages	Disadvantages
• Cheaper and easier to conduct than RCTs and cohort studies	• Significant risk of confounding
• Can be conducted by small teams or individual researchers and can consider multiple exposures	• Difficult to obtain reliable data about exposure of an individual
	• Can be difficult to establish time frames from exposure to disease
• Can often achieve more useful results than cohort studies in rare diseases, particularly where long lag time between exposure and disease	• Causation unlikely to be proved in this type of study
	• Control groups can be difficult to select without bias
• Useful as a preliminary study to consider associations between an exposure and disease	• Risk and incidence cannot be reliably calculated
• Shorter time frame and fewer participants needed than cohort studies	
• Normally no ethical issues in study design	

FIGURE 5.7 Brief summary of the advantages and disadvantages of case-control studies

Odds ratio

The usual outcome of a case-control study is the odds ratio (OR). The odds ratio can approximate to the relative risk with certain criteria being met and you will sometimes see a case-control study reporting its results as relative risk. However, because normally the ratio of cases to controls does not often reflect the ratio of people with and without the outcome of interest in the source population, the odds ratio has to be used instead of relative risk.

The odds ratio looks at the odds within the case group and compares this with the odds within the control group. The odds of an event are the ratio of people with a condition to people without the condition. Odds are calculated by dividing the number with the condition by the number of people without the condition. This is different to probability, which is the number with a condition divided by the total number in the group. The OR is calculated by working out the ratio of events to non-events in the exposed group and dividing this by the ratio of events to non-events in the control group.

To work out the formula for the OR, first a letter from a to d is used to represent each possible outcome, and each letter is used in the formula as shown on the next page.

Odds ratio

	Disease present (cases)	No disease (controls)
Exposure	**a**	**b**
No exposure	**c**	**d**

$$OR = \frac{(a/c)}{(b/d)} = \frac{ad}{bc}$$

Note that $(a/c)/(b/d)$ is the same as ad/bc. This may be useful to remember in an exam situation if you are struggling to work out an answer.

An odds ratio of 1 means there is no association between exposure and outcome. If the OR is less than 1, this indicates that the exposure is protective. You can interpret the OR in two ways, and both are correct. This is best illustrated with an example. If a study looking at smoking and heart disease found an odds ratio of 3.0, this can be interpreted as the odds of someone with heart disease being a smoker is three times greater than those without heart disease *or* that the odds of someone who is a smoker having heart disease is 3.0 times greater than for a non-smoker.

Q 5.19 The following contingency table was constructed after a case-control study was completed showing the number of people who had developed gastrointestinal (GI) cancer after being exposed to chemical X. Calculate the odds ratio for people who have been exposed to chemical X developing GI cancer.

	GI cancer present	No GI cancer	Total
Exposed to X	10	100	110
Not exposed to X	100	200	300
Total	110	300	410

a) 0.1
b) 0.2
c) 1
d) 5
e) 10

The odds ratio for the figures given in the contingency table is calculated as follows:

$$\frac{(a/c)}{(b/d)} = \frac{(10/100)}{(100/200)} = \frac{0.1}{0.5} = 0.2$$

Alternatively:

$$\frac{ad}{bc} = \frac{10 \times 200}{100 \times 100} = \frac{2000}{10\,000} = 0.2$$

The odds ratio is 0.2, therefore the odds of having GI cancer after being exposed to chemical X is 0.2 or 20%. Chemical X appears to be a protective factor against the development of GI cancer. Of the 110 exposed to chemical X only 10 developed GI cancer (10:100 or 1:10), whereas of the 300 people who had not been exposed to chemical X, 100 developed GI cancer (100:200 or 1:2). The odds among those exposed to the chemical are much lower than the odds among those not exposed. Further investigation may be helpful to work out whether there are any confounding factors that may account for this relationship.

Q 5.20 Which of the following is the best definition of a confounder in a case-control study?
a) A factor that causes statistical interpretation to be invalid
b) A variable that is not included in a statistical calculation
c) A factor that relates to both the exposure and the disease and distorts the relationship between them
d) A factor that relates to both the exposure and the disease and makes them more likely to appear to be unrelated
e) A factor that relates to both the exposure and the disease and makes them more likely to appear to be related

The answer to this question is straightforward: confounders can be either positively or negatively correlated to both exposure and the disease and thereby have an impact on the overall result, so the correct definition is C. During study design, attention should be paid to possible confounders (*see* Chapter 3 for more on confounders). It is possible to over-control as well as overlook possible confounders.

CASE SERIES AND CASE REPORTS

A case series is a descriptive study of a group of people who have received the same treatment or who have the same disease. A case report is simply a description of a single person's response to treatment or a case of an unusual illness that warrants particular interest. Case series can obviously be arrived at after several case reports have been made.

These studies cannot directly compare cases with other people who have been treated differently or who do not have the disease in question. This means that there is less opportunity for meaningful statistical analysis: you cannot calculate relative risk or odds ratios, for example. Their usefulness lies partly in helping formulate hypotheses and suggesting possible exposures that may be causal in particular disease processes.

Normally case series are cases identified within a specific time frame, although this time frame varies widely between studies and with extremely rare events it may cover decades. Case series sample the population that have had a particular event occur to them, and normally case series specify a setting or locality as well as the time frame. This can mean that the complete population is included in the sample – that is, every person who has experienced the particular (rare) event within the study time frame and setting is included in the study.

Case series may look at many things but they tend to be best for rare events. Adverse outcomes following, for example, joint replacement surgery in a particular hospital would be a good example of where a case series would be helpful.

Case series could be particularly useful where concerns have been raised and a quick answer is required as to the existence of a possible risk. A good example of this was a case series reported in 1993 that showed that aseptic meningitis was associated with a particular live mumps vaccine (containing the Urabe strain of the virus). This type of vaccine was then withdrawn and an alternative used.* It was found that the risk period fell within a certain time frame (15–35 days) after having the mumps vaccine and a correlation was therefore established.

To be useful a case series needs a clear objective or study question, it needs to set out the time frame of the study, and it needs to set out what inclusion and exclusion criteria have been used. Studies that enrol all eligible patients are more useful than those that only enrol a selection. There should be a high follow-up rate, as any patients lost to follow-up could potentially mean a large difference in the results. Data should, where possible, be collected prospectively.

Ultimately, case series need to demonstrate clinically useful outcomes. It is clear that such studies could easily be used in general practice to consider how

---

* Miller E, Goldacre M, Pugh S, *et al.* Risk of aseptic meningitis after measles, mumps, and rubella vaccine in UK children. *Lancet.* 1993; **341**(8851): 979–82.

treatments are affecting your patients and to form hypotheses that could be tested in more robust studies.

Case reports may be used where something very rare occurs. If such an event occurs, by writing about it and publishing a report other people may reflect on whether they have seen anything similar. Sometimes this may lead to a case series, where it is recognised by others that similar events have occurred. This may be very useful when an apparently new disease occurs due to a mutation in a virus, for example. It may also be useful to explore unique circumstances that led to the rare outcome. These reports are often qualitative in nature and can only include limited descriptive statistics.

Advantages	Disadvantages
• Relatively quick and simple	• Limited in scope and generalisability
• Good for studying rare events	• Inherent bias in selection
• No need for control groups	• Limited conclusions can be drawn

FIGURE 5.8 Brief summary of the advantages and disadvantages of case series and case reports

EXPERT OPINION AND EDITORIALS

We all use expert opinion during our training and subsequent work as qualified GPs. We come into contact with many colleagues with greater knowledge about medical subjects than we ourselves possess. As GPs we look to provide patients with the best care and hence we need to have a broad medical knowledge. Of course, we also need to know about non-medical subjects, such as how to get patients to open up and talk about their emotions.

It is very common for a GP or GP trainee to come into contact with other health professionals who are experts in their field. When someone with a lot of experience and knowledge based on years of training and working in a speciality tells us something, it is understandable that we take that person's words as being valuable and useful. In addition, when we see something that is written down by such a person, it becomes even more powerful – it can be revisited, reread and assimilated more fully and deeply.

Of course if we are told something that reinforces what we already know or think, it is more likely to be accepted as true. This sort of knowledge will often be easily transferred to our everyday practice and influence the decisions we make. We can call upon it easily because it relates to our already held knowledge and beliefs.

Editorials are often written by experts in their field and are a way of summarising the current state of a particular field. They can be very persuasive and are often easier to assimilate than original research articles. They can be based on knowledge of many research studies and therefore they can be very helpful to non-specialists in that field.

However, in the hierarchy of evidence, this type of knowledge comes right at the bottom. Why is this? Because it is opinion rather than evidence and it has not been systematically tested for how true it is. That is why the National Institute for Health and Care Excellence, for example, uses this sort of information but tries to avoid relying on it as much as possible.

Unfortunately, there are many questions in medicine that are unanswered by good-quality studies and there are many areas of medicine where we have to rely on opinion rather than evidence. Where this is the case, we have to be ready to challenge our own preconceptions, assumptions and mistakes and change our practice to reflect the best available evidence. Evidence-based practice grew out of the realisation that many treatments were not based on good-quality evidence and that expert opinion was often incorrect.

Expert opinion needs to be treated with caution. We must be aware that expert opinion will (indeed, should) change over time. However, although expert opinion may be at the bottom of the hierarchy of evidence, it should be acknowledged that we probably use this sort of knowledge a lot in our everyday practice. Where there is lack of evidence we may already be giving the most appropriate treatments, but we need to be aware that we may need to change our practice and this entails knowing where to find the best evidence and how to interpret it.

CONCLUSION

In this chapter we have looked at the different levels in the hierarchy of evidence and discussed the study methods that are included in the hierarchy. We have also looked at the outcome measures for these studies. The hierarchy of evidence is an idealised model and has to be treated as such, but understanding more about the techniques used to conduct research allows a deeper appreciation of both the benefits and the problems with different research methods.

The most important considerations with any research is whether it answers a clinically appropriate question using well-conducted research that tries to avoid bias as much as possible and allows us to assess this by accurately reporting the research methods. This obviously calls for an ability to assess research evidence. Chapter 7 looks at ways of finding and assessing evidence. The next chapter continues looking at quantitative methods but looks at those methods that are commonly used in epidemiology.

CHAPTER 6

Epidemiology

INTRODUCTION

Epidemiology is *the study of the health of populations*. It focuses on the **patterns** of health and disease within a population and tries to identify causative or risk factors. It also looks at the **effects** of health and disease on populations. Epidemiology is the basis for public health interventions and informs population-level policymaking.

Epidemiology takes a broad view of health and disease. It uses all the methods and techniques we have discussed in previous chapters. There are techniques and concepts that are predominantly used in epidemiology and which we will cover in this chapter. For the AKT, you need to have a good grasp of the different concepts used in epidemiology and you also need to be able to perform common calculations, such as sensitivity and specificity.

As GPs we need to be aware of the wider drivers of health and disease in the populations we treat. This is where an understanding of epidemiology becomes invaluable. We use epidemiological data during disease outbreaks in order to understand who is at risk, when and why. For example, during flu outbreaks, it is invaluable to know which sectors of the population are at high risk in order to target vaccination programmes. We also use epidemiological data to help target preventive interventions – for example, encouraging patients to stop smoking, giving whooping cough vaccination to pregnant women, or bowel cancer screening for people aged over 60 (in England and Wales). Epidemiological data tell us which groups are at risk or who will benefit the most from interventions.

Public health is concerned with obtaining the best outcome for the greatest number of people. This is where our everyday practice differs from that of public health practitioners. As GPs we are concerned foremost, but not solely, with the person consulting with us. We need to remember that how we treat one patient has an effect on the population more widely. If we use a very expensive drug to treat one patient, this may decrease the availability of effective and cheap drugs for many other people. We will look at economic evaluation of treatments at the end of this chapter.

ENVIRONMENTAL DETERMINANTS OF HEALTH

The *Applied Knowledge Test Content Guide*, available on the RCGP website, suggests you should be aware of how environmental factors affect health. Here we will consider these alongside primary, secondary and tertiary prevention of disease.

Primary prevention aims to prevent people developing diseases or to protect people from harm. We do a considerable amount of this as GPs – for example, vaccinations and opportunistic lifestyle advice on exercise, weight, alcohol, diet and smoking in order that they may avoid developing diseases such as diabetes and cardiovascular disease. Governments and public health departments are also involved in this, with things like legislation on seatbelt and motorbike helmet use, laws on who can access potentially harmful drugs, health and safety at work legislation and regulations, and public information campaigns.

Secondary prevention covers those interventions after a disease, condition or risk factor occurs but before it has caused any harm. A common example in our work is lifestyle advice and prescribing medication to people who have been diagnosed with impaired fasting glycaemia or hypertension. Finding disease and treating it early can often prevent future harm. This is discussed in the section on screening later in this chapter.

Tertiary prevention is acting after the disease or condition has been diagnosed and has caused harm or symptoms. The aim is to minimise harm from an acute event, improve quality of life and prevent future complications. Examples include treating someone who has had a myocardial infarction with a statin, antiplatelet drug, beta blocker and an ACE inhibitor. If someone is diagnosed with colorectal cancer, that person may have a bowel resection followed by chemotherapy.

Many factors affect people's likelihood of developing disease; some of these are individual factors such as smoking or high alcohol consumption, but many are environmental and without the control of the individual. These environmental factors can be divided into the physical environment and the socio-economic environment. These factors include poverty and poor housing. There are clear links between socio-economic status and risk of many diseases. For example, the risk of many infectious diseases is increased by overcrowding, poor sanitation and poor nutrition, and the outcome is often worse as well.

Often dealing with environmental risk factors can have a greater impact than dealing with the consequences. This is the task of public health professionals, but it is something that GPs should also be aware of and engage with in order to improve the health of our patients. You should be aware of the Black Report of 1980,[*] which concluded that the main cause of health inequality was economic inequality. The Acheson Report of 1998[†] set out suggestions for policies to tackle growing health inequalities in Britain. A further review, published in 2010 by Professor Sir Michael Marmot,[‡] built on these earlier reports and pointed to the wider benefits of tackling health inequalities.

However, there remains much inequality in health outcomes across Britain. The average life expectancy in the most-deprived areas is 9.2 years less than the life expectancy in the least-deprived areas of England.[§] The gap is even bigger if the most-deprived areas of Scotland are considered as well. In the face of such statistics we feel powerless, but good healthcare is vital for these most-deprived areas. The 'inverse care law' was proposed by Dr Julian Tudor Hart in 1971; this suggests that the areas most in need of good healthcare are the least likely to receive it.[¶]

Let us now turn to look at some questions covering epidemiological topics.

Q 6.1   From the table, choose the correct definition for each of the following words.

a) Specificity

b) Sensitivity

c) Prevalence

d) Positive predictive value

e) Incidence

1) The total number of cases within a population at a particular time point

2) How likely a person who tests positive is to have the condition being tested for

3) How good a test is at detecting the condition of interest in those people with it

4) The number of new cases of a disorder developing over a given time within a specified population

5) How good a test is at excluding the condition of interest in those people who do not have it

* Department of Health and Social Security. *Inequalities in Health: report of a research working group* [the Black Report]. London: DHSS; 1980.

† Department of Health. *Independent Inquiry into Inequalities in Health Report* [the Acheson Report]. London: The Stationery Office; 1998.

‡ Marmot M. *Fair Society, Healthy Lives: the Marmot Review; strategic review of health inequalities in England post-2010*. London: Marmot Review; 2010.

§ Office for National Statistics. *Statistical Bulletin: inequality in healthy life expectancy at birth by national deciles of area deprivation: England, 2009-11*. London: Office for National Statistics; 2014.

¶ Tudor Hart J. The inverse care law. *Lancet*. 1971; **297**(7696): 405–12.

Q 6.2 A clinical commissioning group requires information to enable it to plan services for people with lung cancer. It wishes to know the typical length of service provision that is needed for this group of patients. Which of the following options would be the most helpful measure in this situation?

a) A case fatality
b) Incidence
c) Mortality
d) Median survival
e) Prevalence

Q 6.3 Use each abbreviation or phrase in the following list to complete the positions A–J in the contingency table provided.

1) TN
2) FP
3) Positive predictive value
4) Disease absent
5) Positive test result

6) FN
7) Negative predictive value
8) Sensitivity
9) Disease present
10) Specificity

(TP = true positive, FP = false positive, FN = false negative, TN = true negative)

Contingency table	A	B	
C	TP	D	E
Negative test result	F	G	H
	I	J	

Q 6.4 Which of the following measures would be most helpful in estimating the rate at which a viral infection affects people living in a particular area?

a) Case fatality
b) Incidence
c) Median survival
d) Mortality
e) Prevalence

INCIDENCE

The terms incidence and prevalence are often confused when being learnt or recalled. *Incidence is the number of **new** cases of a disease or condition in a particular population starting in a given period of time.* This would normally be expressed as a rate of new cases in relation to a population. So, it may be expressed as per

10 000, per 100 000, or any other figure. The denominator varies and will be chosen based on the total size of the population and in relation to other diseases, if comparisons are being made. Pay attention to the denominator: there is obviously a tenfold difference between 5 in 10 000 and 5 in 100 000, and this will alter how a particular disease may be understood and treated.

Incidence does not have to refer to diseases; it can also refer to risk factors or behaviour. For example, the incidence of smoking in teenagers can provide us with a picture of whether smoking rates are affected by public health information programmes. If the incidence of smoking goes down while an intervention is in progress, then this suggests that intervention is working.

Note also that the rate is in a given period of time. There is a big difference between 50 in a month per 10 000 and 50 in 5 years per 10 000. Be aware that the incidence may vary over time and this will not be obvious unless the incidence is given for suitable periods of time. For example, the incidence of flu cases will normally be much higher in winter than in summer. Therefore, it makes sense to give the incidence figures for flu for a relatively short time frame such as a week and to show how the rate compares with previous weeks.

Incidence can be very useful for determining disease aetiology. This can be done by seeking out which risk factors have changed when incidence varies, so that important aetiological factors are identified. In order to fully understand a disease process, we will also need to know how widespread the disease is and for how long the disease affects people. This is prevalence, which is discussed further later in this chapter.

There are two commonly used formulas for calculating incidence: the first is for incidence rate and the second is for incidence proportion. The formula for working out incidence is simply the number of new cases divided by the specified population for the time frame over which the data are collected.

Incidence rate

$$\frac{\text{number of new cases starting during specified time interval}}{\text{average population during specified time interval}}$$

Sometimes the denominator for incidence rate is the sum of the observed person-years.

Incidence proportion

$$\frac{\text{number of new cases during specified time interval}}{\text{population at start of time period}}$$

These are normally given as a rate or proportion for a specified population, such as per 100 000 or per 10 000.

Actually, there is not a lot of difference between the two if the population is relatively large and stable, but where there is a transient population, or high mortality rates in a small population, this distinction can be important. It is useful to remember, however, that there is a difference between a rate and a proportion.

Q 6.5 An epidemiological study finds that within an English county population of 1 000 000, there are 135 people newly diagnosed with leukaemia over a 1-year period. What is the incidence of leukaemia for this population?
a) 13.5 per 100 000 per year
b) 13.5 per 10 000 per year
c) 7.25 per 100 000 per year
d) 135 per 100 000 per year
e) 1.35 per 1000 per year

Q 6.6 The same county had 1320 new cases of lung cancer over 2 years. What is the annual incidence proportion of lung cancer for this population?
a) 1320 per 100 000
b) 660 per 100 000
c) 66 per 10 000
d) 1320 per 1 000 000
e) 6.6 per 10 000

In Questions 6.5 and 6.6 we have a population of one million. There are 135 new cases of leukaemia in the population of a million people in a single year, so the incidence proportion of leukaemia per 100 000 is calculated as follows.

$$\frac{135}{1\,000\,000} = 0.000\,135 \text{ per year}$$
$$0.000\,135 \times 100\,000 = 13.5 \text{ per } 100\,000$$

This is the same as 135 per million or 1.35 per 10 000.

The number of new lung cancer cases in Question 6.6 is for 2 years; therefore, for an annual incidence rate you have to divide the total number of cases of lung cancer by 2. This gives 660 per million per year. This is the same as 66 per 100 000 or 6.6 per 10 000.

Q 6.7 In a population of a county in England with a population of one million, there are 1600 intravenous drug users. Among these intravenous drug users, 140 had new infections of hepatitis C in 2012. What is the incidence of hepatitis C in that year for intravenous drug users in this county?

a) 140 per 1000 per year
b) 7.3 per 100 per month
c) 87.5 per 1000 per year
d) 87.5 per 10 000 per year
e) 8.75 per 1000 per year

This is slightly more complicated, simply because you have to work with slightly more awkward numbers. To work this out, you divide the number of cases (140) by the population (1600, not one million, as you are interested in the incidence among intravenous drug users only) and then divide by the time (1 year).

$$\frac{140}{1600} = 0.0875 \quad 0.0875 \times 1000 = 87.5$$

This is 87.5 per 1000 per year. The incidence per month would be 7.3 per 1000 $(87.5/12 = 7.3)$.

PREVALENCE

Prevalence is often compared to a snapshot. *Prevalence is the proportion of cases in a given population at a given time.* This, like incidence, can refer to both diseases and other factors such as smoking or pregnancy. Like incidence, prevalence should be given as a ratio with a suitable denominator; knowing the number of cases per 10 000 or per 100 000 helps in commissioning healthcare.

Prevalence

$$\frac{\text{total number of people with a condition at a given time}}{\text{population}}$$

The time frame for prevalence should be specified, as prevalence can change over time. A disease such as flu will normally have high incidence and prevalence only for a short time in the winter in Britain. Because flu is a relatively short illness, the prevalence will be closely related to incidence. Obviously, with flu you would want to know the prevalence at a given point (point prevalence) or over a short time frame (period prevalence). However, with other prolonged illnesses or chronic disease, you may be interested in the (period) prevalence over a much greater time frame, such as a year or decade.

Sometimes it is helpful to know what the prevalence is over a lifetime; for example, the lifetime prevalence of a particular vaccination – the proportion of the population who have had the vaccination at any point in their lifetime. This would provide a good idea of whether the population would have herd immunity from the disease that was vaccinated against.

The practicalities of collecting data mean that both incidence and prevalence are often estimates based on samples. In some cases, because of practical and financial restraints, they are collected over an extended period of time – this can of course affect the results if the prevalence of the condition being studied changes rapidly.

Q 6.8   In an English city of 200 000 there are a total of 610 people with flu during a 1-week period in February. What is the prevalence?
a) 610 per 100 000 per week
b) 0.061%
c) 305 per 100 000 per week
d) 0.035%
e) You can't work out prevalence from the figures given

Q 6.9   This table shows the prevalence of oesophageal cancer over 1, 5 and 10 years for an English region. Which of the following options will affect the prevalence rates given in the table? There may be one or more correct answers.

One-year prevalence: 8.3 per 100 000 age-standardised population

Five-year prevalence: 16.6 per 100 000 age-standardised population

Ten-year prevalence: 19.3 per 100 000 age-standardised population

a) Improvements in treatment over the 10 years studied
b) Incidence of oesophageal cancer
c) Early detection of oesophageal cancer
d) More elderly people in the population of interest
e) Survival rates for oesophageal cancer

Question 6.8 is straightforward: you have a population of 200 000 and 610 cases; therefore, dividing both numerator and denominator by 2 gives 305 per 100 000. It is important to state the time frame as well, because this would have a significant impact on prevalence.

The question on oesophageal cancer needs an understanding of what affects prevalence. Obviously, higher incidence combined with increased survival rates would lead to greater prevalence. Having earlier detection and improved treatment affects prevalence, because both of these will impact on the survival rate. Detecting cancer earlier often means there is a better chance of successful radical treatment. Having more elderly people in a population is controlled for by using age-standardised rates, so this would not affect the prevalence rates of oesophageal cancer.

SCREENING PROGRAMMES

Screening looks for disease in people from a defined population who are apparently well, with no signs of disease. If disease is picked up early, then people can be treated early. This approach holds the promise of saving lives and potentially saving healthcare systems money as well. However, as Wilson and Jungner pointed out, 'in theory … screening is an admirable method for combatting disease … [but] in practice, there are snags'.[*] They came up with their widely known 10 principles for screening programmes in order to try to avoid some of those snags (*see* Figure 6.1).

---

1. The condition sought should be an important health problem.
2. There should be an accepted treatment for patients with recognised disease.
3. Facilities for diagnosis and treatment should be available.
4. There should be a recognisable latent or early symptomatic stage.
5. There should be a suitable test or examination.
6. The test should be acceptable to the population.
7. The natural history of the condition, including development from latent to declared disease, should be adequately understood.
8. There should be an agreed policy on whom to treat as patients.
9. The cost of case-finding (including diagnosis and treatment of patients diagnosed) should be economically balanced in relation to possible expenditure on medical care as a whole.
10. Case-finding should be a continuing process and not a 'once and for all' project.

FIGURE 6.1 Wilson and Jungner criteria for screening programmes[*]

These criteria have been updated over the years since they were originally published. The World Health Organization has looked at the many refinements or alterations suggested, and has come up with modified criteria (*see* Figure 6.2).

---

[*] Wilson JMG, Jungner G. *Principles and Practice of Screening for Disease*. Public Health Paper No. 34. Geneva: World Health Organization; 1968.

1. The screening programme should respond to a recognised need.
2. The objectives of screening should be defined at the outset.
3. There should be a defined target population.
4. There should be scientific evidence of screening programme effectiveness.
5. The programme should integrate education, testing, clinical services and programme management.
6. There should be quality assurance, with mechanisms to minimise potential risks of screening.
7. The programme should ensure informed choice, confidentiality and respect for autonomy.
8. The programme should promote equity and access to screening for the entire target population.
9. Programme evaluation should be planned from the outset.
10. The overall benefits of screening should outweigh the harm.

FIGURE 6.2 Modified Wilson and Jungner criteria[*]

The National Health Service has several screening programmes, including antenatal screening, newborn screening, mammography and bowel cancer screening. There is controversy over some of these programmes, because studies have shown that more harm than benefit can be caused.[†] Because screening can cause harm as well as provide benefits, there needs to be formal assessment of any existing or proposed screening programme. Some of the methods to do this are discussed next.

SENSITIVITY AND SPECIFICITY

These are a couple of terms that are also often confused. They are often used in epidemiology, particularly when evaluating screening tests. Essentially, sensitivity and specificity are ways of evaluating a test in terms of how good it is at identifying both people with the disease and people without the disease. The ideal would be to have values of 100% – that is, everyone with the disease is identified as having the disease and everyone without the disease is identified as not having it.

Interestingly, although sensitivity and specificity are concepts that are often taught to undergraduate medical students, they are not particularly helpful in diagnostic medicine. They are not measures that apply to individual patients: you cannot work out how likely someone is to have a disease or not based on sensitivity and specificity. They are useful for evaluating population-level tests,

---

[*] Andermann A, Blancquaert I, Beauchamp S, *et al.* Revisiting Wilson and Jungner in the genomic age: a review of screening criteria over the past 40 years. *Bull World Health Organ.* 2008; **86**(4): 317–19.

[†] See, for example, Miller AB, Wall C, Baines CJ, *et al.* Twenty five year follow-up for breast cancer incidence and mortality of the Canadian National Breast Screening Study: randomised screening trial. *BMJ.* 2014; **348**: g366.

also known as screening tests. To evaluate the probability of a patient having a disease based on a test result requires predictive values or likelihood ratios, which are discussed later in this chapter.

From practical experience, doctors understand that tests are rarely, if ever, completely sensitive and specific. Even those tests considered to be gold standards will have an element of error in them. Tests that appear to be very accurate or precise (*see* Chapter 2) can sometimes be unhelpful and often even common tests (think of X-rays and scans) need specialist interpretation. Some tests are misleading because of false positive or false negative results – this can be the start of the wrong line of enquiry or treatment or non-treatment. All tests should be approached with caution and this is where sensitivity and specificity are helpful to quantify the usefulness of a test.

The rates of true and false negatives and positives are often worked out by comparing a test with the gold standard. Completing other types of study based on populations and in particular on post-mortems can be helpful to validate how accurate the gold standard is.

Sensitivity is how good a test is at detecting people with the condition. A highly sensitive test is one that does not miss many cases of disease: it is sensitive to the disease. This is found by dividing the number of people with the condition and whom the test identifies as having the condition (true positives) by the total number of people with the condition.

Sensitivity

$$\frac{\text{true positives}}{\text{number of people with the condition}}$$

Specificity is how good a test is at excluding those people without the condition. A highly specific test is one that does not have many false positives: it is specific to the disease. This is found by dividing the number of people without the condition and whom the test identifies as not having the condition (true negatives) by the total number of people without the condition.

Specificity

$$\frac{\text{true negatives}}{\text{number of people without the condition}}$$

In order to be able to calculate sensitivity and specificity, the first step is to construct a contingency table. For evaluating sensitivity and specificity, Figure 6.3 has the number of positive tests split into true and false positives and the number of negatives split into true and false negatives. The same method can also be used to calculate predictive values.

	Condition present	Condition absent
Test positive	TP	FP
Test negative	FN	TN

FIGURE 6.3 A contingency table for calculating sensitivity and specificity (TP = true positive, FP = false positive, FN = false negative, TN = true negative)

Given Figure 6.3, we can work out the formulas for sensitivity and specificity. Sensitivity is the number of true positives divided by the total number of people with the condition. From Figure 6.3, you can see that if you add together the true positives and the false negatives, you will have the total number of people with the disease; therefore, the denominator is TP + FN.

Sensitivity

$$\frac{\text{true positives}}{\text{true positives} + \text{false negatives}} = \frac{\text{TP}}{\text{TP} + \text{FN}}$$

Similarly, you can work out specificity by dividing the true negatives by the total number of people without the condition. The total of people without the disease is the false positives plus the true negatives.

Specificity

$$\frac{\text{true negatives}}{\text{false positives} + \text{true negatives}} = \frac{\text{TN}}{\text{FP} + \text{TN}}$$

If you look at the contingency table you can see that you are working down the columns. Hence, sensitivity is calculated using the data in the first column, and specificity by using the data in the second column. It is possible for the data to be presented with the condition present or absent in the first column and test positive or negative in the second and third columns. Make sure you check the table is set out in the way you are used to working; if it is not, change it so that it is, to avoid making mistakes.

When evaluating a test, it is important to look at both the sensitivity and the specificity in order to ascertain how useful that test is. However, there are very definite limits to their usefulness, a major limitation being that prevalence of a condition is not reflected in sensitivity and specificity. This can lead to problems: where a condition has a very high prevalence this will mean that even very high sensitivity and specificity may result in large absolute numbers of false positives and negatives.

A test with 100% sensitivity is limited in its usefulness if it has a low specificity. Consider a test that has 100% sensitivity but only 50% specificity; the test will identify everyone with the disease but it will also be positive for one in two people without the disease. This will mean you have a potentially large number of people who have a positive test but who will not have the condition of interest. If the disease is relatively uncommon, you may have a very large number of positive results but only a very small number of those will actually truly have the disease. This test would be useful for ruling out a disease where it is negative.

Conversely, a test with very high specificity but low sensitivity would be useful for identifying people with disease. However, it would also lead to a number of tests with false negative results and therefore people with the disease would not be identified as having it. It is clear that we need other ways of evaluating a test in order to avoid these pitfalls.

Q 6.10 The results from a study evaluating the prostate-specific antigen (PSA) blood test as a screening test for prostate cancer are shown in the following table. These results assume that a value >3 ng/mL is positive. Calculate the sensitivity and specificity from these results. In addition, calculate the prevalence of the disease in those studied.[*]

	Prostate cancer present	Prostate cancer absent
PSA test positive	118	26
PSA test negative	82	174

Answers:

Sensitivity	Specificity	Prevalence

---

[*] Data in Questions 6.10 and 6.11 based on a paper by Benny Holmström *et al.* (Holmström B, Johansson M, Bergh A, *et al.* Prostate specific antigen for early detection of prostate cancer: longitudinal study. *BMJ.* 2009; **339**: b3537.)

Q **6.11** The same study is completed in a population with a very different prevalence of prostate cancer. Work out the sensitivity and specificity and then work out the prevalence of prostate cancer in this study.

	Prostate cancer present	Prostate cancer absent
PSA test positive	59	1287
PSA test negative	41	8613

Answers:

Sensitivity	Specificity	Prevalence

To work out sensitivity, we divide the number of true positives by the total number of people in the study with the disease (as proven by a prostate biopsy – the gold standard for diagnosis of prostate cancer).

For Question 6.10 this gives us:

$$\frac{118}{118 + 82} = \frac{118}{200} = 0.59$$

Likewise, to work out specificity we divide the true negatives by the total of people without the disease:

$$\frac{174}{174 + 26} = \frac{174}{200} = 0.87$$

The sensitivity is 0.59 or 59% and the specificity is 0.87 or 87%.

To work out the prevalence, you divide the number of confirmed cases by the total population. In this case you have a total population of 400 (TP + FP + TN + FN), and out of that population, 200 people have confirmed prostate cancer. This gives a prevalence of 50%. This is unlikely to occur.

The answers to Question 6.11 are worked out in the same way.

$$\frac{59}{59 + 41} = \frac{59}{100} = 0.59$$

The sensitivity is 59%, the same as in the previous question.

$$\frac{8613}{8613 + 1287} = \frac{8613}{9900} = 0.87$$

This gives the same specificity as well: 87%.

So the sensitivity and specificity are the same in both the sets of results given here. However, the prevalence is very different. For Question 6.11, the total number of people with prostate cancer is 100 and the total number of men in the population is 9900. Therefore, the prevalence is slightly more than 1%.

This demonstrates how knowing the sensitivity and specificity does not tell the full story about screening tests. The actual results need to be interpreted in line with having an idea of how prevalent a condition is. Given the second set of figures, if you screen 10 000 men with a cut-off for a positive PSA chosen to be 3 ng/mL, you will have 59 true positive results and 1287 false positive results. Only about 4.4% of the positive results will be in men with prostate cancer (*see* the next section on positive predictive values). In addition you will have 41 men who are falsely reassured with a negative result but who will have prostate cancer.

We obviously need more than just sensitivity and specificity in order to evaluate screening tests. We look at likelihood ratios later in this chapter – these are another helpful tool for working out how useful a screening test is. First, though, we look at positive and negative predictive values.

POSITIVE AND NEGATIVE PREDICTIVE VALUES

Sensitivity and specificity are measures of the effectiveness of a test at a population level. That is, they tell you how likely someone with a condition is going to have a correct screening test result. Predictive values are more helpful when faced with an individual patient. The question that a clinician wants to answer is 'Given a test result, how likely is this patient to have condition X?' Predictive values can help answer this question.

The positive predictive value (PPV) is how likely someone who tests positive is to actually have the condition being tested for. This means that you need to only include the people who have tested positive in the calculation. You divide the number of true positives by the total number of positive tests. The larger the positive predictive value, the lower the number of false positives the test will result in.

The formula for the positive predictive value is therefore:

PPV

$$\frac{\text{true positives}}{\text{true positives} + \text{false positives}} = \frac{\text{TP}}{\text{TP} + \text{FP}}$$

Note: this is not the ratio of true positives to false positives, because the denominator for this calculation includes all the positive tests. This is actually the probability of a positive test being correct. If, however, you consider the ratio of correct positives to incorrect positives, that gives you the odds of the test being correct.

A *negative predictive value (NPV) is how likely someone who tests negative is to not have the condition being tested for.* This means that the higher the negative predictive value, the more likely someone who tests negative will not have the condition.

The formula for the negative predictive value is therefore:

$$NPV$$

$$\frac{\text{true negatives}}{\text{true negatives} + \text{false negatives}} = \frac{TN}{TN + FN}$$

With sensitivity and specificity, you were working down the columns of the contingency table, looking at whether the condition was present or absent. With predictive values, you are working across the rows, looking at whether the test is positive or negative. The contingency table can be extended, as shown here, to remind you of what each of these four measures is measuring and how they are calculated.

	Condition present	Condition absent	
Test positive	TP	FP	PPV
Test negative	FN	TN	NPV
	Sensitivity	Specificity	

FIGURE 6.4 A contingency table showing the direction in which you work for sensitivity, specificity, positive predictive value (PPV) and negative predictive value (NPV)

Q 6.12

Work out the PPV and NPV for the data presented in Questions 6.10 and 6.11. Give your answers as a percentage to one decimal place and record them in the following table.

Data from Question 6.10

	Prostate cancer present	Prostate cancer absent
PSA test positive	118	26
PSA test negative	82	174

Data from Question 6.11

	Prostate cancer present	Prostate cancer absent
PSA test positive	59	1287
PSA test negative	41	8613

Answers:

	PPV	NPV
Data from Question 6.10		
Data from Question 6.11		

If we work out the PPV and NPV for the population in Question 6.10, where the population is 400 and the prevalence of prostate cancer is 50%, we get the following results.

For PPV:

$$\frac{118}{118 + 26} = \frac{118}{144} = 0.819 = 81.9\%$$

For NPV:

$$\frac{174}{174 + 82} = \frac{174}{256} = 0.679 = 67.9\%$$

For the data in Question 6.11 with a population of 10 000 and a prostate cancer prevalence of 1%, we find the PPV is:

$$\frac{59}{59 + 1287} = \frac{59}{1346} = 0.0438 = 4.4\%$$

The NPV is:

$$\frac{8613}{8613 + 41} = \frac{8613}{8654} = 0.995 = 99.5\%$$

This suggests that the PSA test as presented in Question 6.11 is helpful when you have a negative test – it is unlikely that the person in front of you will have a false negative result (in this case, that means a person with a PSA of <3 ng/mL will be unlikely to have prostate cancer).

You can see that the PPV and NPV change when prevalence changes, even though the sensitivity and specificity remain the same. As disease prevalence increases, so too does the positive predictive value. The negative predictive value decreases as prevalence of the disease increases. This means that a positive test is more likely to be correct when the disease is more prevalent, and a negative test is more likely to be correct when the disease is less prevalent.

Positive and negative predictive values are helpful for determining how good a test is at establishing whether a person does or does not have a condition. Sometimes you need to rule people out, in which case the negative predictive value is most helpful. A good example of this would be the first part of a two-part screening test: you first identify those at higher risk by using a test with a high NPV and then use a second test (often more complicated, dangerous and/or expensive) to identify those with the condition. An example of this would be using a faecal occult blood test to screen for bowel cancer followed by a colonoscopy.

The probability, before the test, of someone having the disease is the same as the prevalence of that disease in the population from which the person is drawn. If a disease has 5% prevalence within the studied population, it is reasonable to conclude, before any testing, that 5% of the tests will be positive. This is known as the *prior probability* of disease. The predictive values give a revised estimate of the probability of someone having or not having the disease, given his or her test results. This is known as the *posterior probability*. One way of assessing how useful a test is would be to compare the prior and posterior probabilities.

Remember that for rare diseases, a positive test is more likely to be incorrect and a negative test is more likely to be correct. This applies even when a test has high sensitivity and specificity. This is a fundamental problem for screening programmes – limiting a test to those who have already been assessed as likely to have a disease will make the test more helpful. This is useful to remember in our everyday practice when we decide to order some tests because we are not sure what is going on – such tests are much less helpful than ordering tests based on a thorough history and examination which then suggest a particular disease needs to be considered likely.

Because predictive values are affected by prevalence, they can only be estimated from studies that are population based rather than individual based. Case-control studies can be helpful for predicting sensitivity and specificity but not predictive values. A cross-sectional study will enable predictive values to be worked out. Given this, it is important that predictive values are applied to a population with a similar prevalence of disease as that in the original study.

LIKELIHOOD RATIOS

Likelihood ratios are not affected by the prevalence of a condition and focus on what a test result means for an individual. *They compare the probability of a test result if the patient has the condition, with the probability of the same result if the patient does not have the condition.* They are applicable to individual patients and this makes them very useful. Indeed, they are more useful than sensitivity, specificity or predictive values when a clinician is considering the test result for a particular patient. However, they are not often used in clinical practice, probably because a little bit of calculation or reference to a nomogram is required. This section and the following section on pre- and post-test probabilities make use of Bayes' theorem. This enables prior knowledge and the result of a test to be combined to give us the probability of a particular outcome.

The main advantage of likelihood ratios is that they can be used to help a clinician evaluate a test result for an individual patient. It only makes sense to order the test because you have a strong suspicion that a particular disease affects the patient. The test chosen may rule a disease in or it may rule a disease out (for example, a negative D-dimer test virtually rules out a deep vein thrombosis or pulmonary embolism, if correctly used).

Likelihood ratios combine sensitivity and specificity. They are related to the pre- and post-test probabilities of having a disease, discussed further in the next section. Likelihood ratios are split up into the likelihood ratio for a positive test (LR+) and the likelihood ratio for a negative test (LR−).

The general formula for a likelihood ratio is as follows.

Likelihood ratio

$$\frac{\text{probability of finding in patients with disease}}{\text{probability of same finding in patients without disease}}$$

There are two formulas for likelihood ratios: one for negative and one for positive. They can be derived in several ways but commonly they are derived from sensitivity and specificity. Calculating the LR from sensitivity and specificity is probably the easiest way to remember the formulas.

The formula for the *likelihood ratio for a positive test result* is as follows.

Likelihood ratio for a positive test result

$$\frac{\text{sensitivity}}{1 - \text{specificity}}$$

The formula for the *likelihood ratio for a negative test result* is as follows.

Likelihood ratio for a negative test result

$$\frac{1 - \text{sensitivity}}{\text{specificity}}$$

An LR greater than 1 indicates that the test result is associated with the presence of the condition, whereas an LR of less than 1 indicates that the test result is associated with the absence of the condition. If the LR equals 1, then there is no diagnostic value of the test result, as the probability of the condition being present is the same as it being absent. The further away from 1 the results are, the greater the likelihood of disease being present or absent. Values above 10 and below 0.1 are *generally* taken to provide strong evidence to confirm or refute a diagnosis, but caution should still be exercised in very rare conditions.

Note that this holds true for both positive and negative likelihood ratios. If a negative likelihood ratio has a value of greater than 1, a negative result is more likely to occur in people with the disease of interest than in people without that disease. If a positive likelihood ratio has a value greater than 1, a positive test is more likely to occur in people with the disease of interest. Again this *generally* holds true where the disease is common but caution needs to be exercised with rarer diseases.

Q **6.13** From the following table for the PSA test that we have used before, work out the likelihood ratios for both positive and negative test results and record your answers below.

Data from Question 6.11

	Prostate cancer present	Prostate cancer absent
PSA test positive	59	1287
PSA test negative	41	8613

Remember you already know the sensitivity and specificity from the previous questions.

Answers:

Likelihood ratio for a positive result	Likelihood ratio for a negative result

From these PSA data, we know that the sensitivity is 59% and the specificity is 87%. If we use the likelihood ratio formulas given above, we have to write these as a decimal – that is, 0.59 and 0.87 (alternatively we can use percentages by using 100 in the equations rather than 1).

For a positive PSA test result, the likelihood ratio is:

$$\frac{\text{sensitivity}}{1 - \text{specificity}} = \frac{0.59}{1 - 0.87} = 4.54$$

A value of 10 would suggest strong evidence for the condition being present (this figure of 4.54 is not very close to 10). Remember this result is for a PSA value of >3 ng/mL.

For a negative test result, the likelihood ratio is:

$$\frac{1 - \text{sensitivity}}{\text{specificity}} = \frac{1 - 0.59}{0.87} = 0.47$$

This is not very close to the value of 0.1, the value that would be considered to be strong evidence for ruling out the condition. This result is for a PSA value of <3 ng/mL, because that is considered our cut-off between a positive or negative test for the particular sensitivity and specificity we are using. Remember, that sensitivity and specificity change depending on the chosen cut-off value of the PSA test.

Also remember that likelihood ratios can be used for individual patients and they are not affected by prevalence. The interpretation of these tests is also intuitive: the smaller the negative likelihood ratio, the less likely the condition; the greater the positive likelihood ratio, the greater the likelihood of disease. Once you are aware of the likelihood ratio for a particular test result, you can apply it to other patients. However, to fully understand how these ratios are helpful for individual patients, we need to consider pre- and post-test probability.

PRE- AND POST-TEST PROBABILITY

We know that diagnostic tests are rarely 100% accurate; there is a chance of a false positive and a chance of a false negative. In order to quantify an individual's chance of disease we can use likelihood ratios alongside an estimate of his or her pre-test probability of having the disease.

Predictive values refer to the likelihood (*see* Chapter 2 and Glossary) of testing positive or negative for a disease in a control or study **group**. Post-test probability refers to the likelihood of an **individual** testing positive or negative. The pre-test probability of having a disease can be considered to be roughly the same as the prevalence of that disease within the population being studied. This will be modified based on a clinical history and examination. The estimate of pre-test probability is therefore based on the clinician's experience and local prevalence data. Pre-test probabilities have been calculated and published for some conditions; therefore, a search for relevant literature can be helpful if needing to know a pre-test probability (*see* Chapter 7).

If the prevalence of a condition is low, say 1%, in a population it would be expected that anyone chosen at random from that population will have a similar likelihood of having that condition. Therefore, you would assume their likelihood of having that condition to be around 1%. However, if they have signs and symptoms of that condition and are presenting to a healthcare professional, then they become part of another population with a very different prevalence of the condition. For example, a patient presenting with acute loin pain and haematuria is far more likely to have renal calculi than someone chosen at random from the larger population of an area.

Choosing a test to be performed should be based on the idea that you will significantly alter the probability of a particular disease, therefore making it easier to rule a particular condition in or out. Assuming it is a helpful, appropriate test, if the test is negative it should decrease the probability of disease, and likewise if it is positive, it should increase the probability of the disease.

The probability after the test result is known as, not surprisingly, the *post-test probability*. It is the post-test probability that is most helpful – as clinicians we want to know whether a diagnosis is likely or not. Because it is rare for post-test probability to be either 0% or 100%, a diagnosis will not be made with certainty but this may help in deciding the next step for either further investigation or treatment. Doing another test will further alter the post-test probability and may or may not make a particular diagnosis more likely.

Combining the pre-test probability with the likelihood ratio for a positive or negative test will give the post-test probability. The calculation for post-test probability involves odds and probabilities, so it becomes too complex to easily apply during a consultation. There are easier ways of working out the post-test probability based on using a nomogram.

Fagan's nomogram has pre-test probability on the first line, followed by the likelihood ratio and then the post-test probability. To find out the post-test probability, you draw a straight line through the pre-test probability and likelihood ratio and extend it through to the post-test probability line, giving a reasonably accurate estimation of the post-test probability.

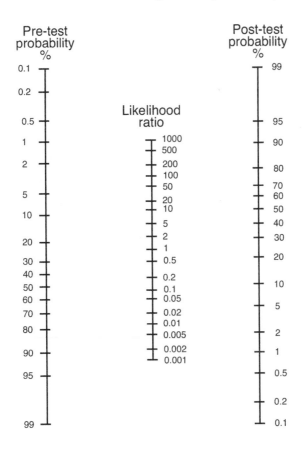

FIGURE 6.5 Fagan's nomogram

Q 6.14 Using the PSA data that we have used throughout this chapter, and with reference to a nomogram, work out the likelihood that a patient has prostate cancer if he has a PSA >3 ng/mL, with a likelihood ratio of 4.54. The pre-test probability, based on a full history and clinical examination including digital rectal examination, is estimated to be 50%, largely because of a suspicious-feeling prostate and the patient being aged 70. Write your answer in the box provided.

To work out the post-test probability of prostate cancer in our 70-year-old man with a PSA result >3 ng/mL and a suspicious digital rectal examination, we take the pre-test probability of 50% and draw a straight line through the likelihood ratio value of 4.54 and extend it to the post-test probability line. It can be seen that this gives us a post-test probability of around 80%. This estimation is good enough for us to be able to make a decision upon our next step for this patient. We can discuss and share a management plan, which may include referral for prostate biopsy if that is what the patient wishes to do. However, the patient may decide he wants to take another approach, based on his outlook or other health problems.

MEASURES OF MORTALITY

Q 6.15 Match the definitions

a) Neonatal mortality rate

b) Infant mortality rate

c) Child mortality rate

d) Mortality rate

e) Survival rate

1) The number of deaths in a specified population in a specified time

2) The percentage of people alive at a specified time after diagnosis

3) The annual number of deaths among children aged 1–4 years

4) The annual number of deaths among children aged under 1 year

5) The annual number of deaths among babies younger than 28 days old

The *mortality rate normally refers to the number of deaths in a specified population.* This is normally reported related both to the size of that population and to a specified period of time. For example, the death rate in the UK during the first quarter of 2013 was 10.2 per thousand. The actual number of deaths registered was 160 900 but this is then divided by the total population. Mortality rates can look at total mortality or they may be concerned with mortality from a particular illness or group of illnesses.

Knowing the mortality rate for a particular disease is useful for public health officials who need to respond to disease outbreaks. For an individual patient, knowing the mortality rate can be useful when discussing treatment options. Of course, that depends on a sensitive discussion rather than a crude presentation of facts.

Consider how a patient diagnosed with prostate cancer may find it helpful to discuss 5-, 10- or 20-year mortality or *survival rates. Survival rates are often presented as percentages of people alive at a given interval after diagnosis.* This is often used when discussing cancer diagnoses. It gives a crude idea of how long a patient may be expected to live for. However, it is not directly applicable to an individual patient – it is applicable to everyone with the disease. This means that for an individual, his or her survival could be very different from the average for people with the same disease. This could be due to stage at presentation, co-morbidities, improved treatments or other factors that are unique to the individual, such as response to treatment.

One way of trying to make survival rates more accurate is to compare a group of people with the disease of interest and similar people without the disease. For example, if a type of slowly progressive cancer mainly affects relatively old people, they may die of other causes and not from that cancer. *Relative survival is calculated by dividing the survival rate after diagnosis of the disease being considered, by the survival rate observed in a similar population without the disease.* The latter group should be matched as closely as possible, so it may be matched for gender, age, location, social class and smoking status, for example.

Cause-specific survival is different to relative survival in that it removes people who die of other causes than the one of interest from the population. So, if a cohort of people with prostate cancer is followed, then anyone who dies from other causes would be considered to reduce the population size but not affect the survival rate for people with prostate cancer.

Mortality rates can be difficult to compare between groups, and particularly countries, when the demographics of those groups vary considerably. An area with a higher number of elderly people would be expected to have a higher mortality rate than an area with fewer elderly people. Removing the effect of age by calculating age-specific death rates and relating this to the number of people in that age group in each location gives a way of comparing mortality rates across differing populations. This is an *age-standardised mortality rate.* It is possible to use standardisation for factors other than age if required.

Life expectancy is an estimate of how long a newborn baby will live based on current age-specific mortality rates. Again this obviously does not apply to an individual very well, but it can be thought of as the expected average age at death for a cohort of people.

The **child mortality rate** normally refers to the annual number of deaths in children aged between 1 and 4 years given as a rate per 1000 children in that age group. The **infant mortality rate** applies to children younger than 1 year of age given as a rate per 1000 live births in that year. The **neonatal mortality rate** applies to deaths in infants younger than 28 days of age.

The **case fatality rate** is also known as the fatality rate. It is the number of deaths due to a particular condition, compared with the number of people who contract the condition, over the course of a disease or condition. This is often used for diseases with limited time courses, such as outbreaks of acute infections. This differs from the mortality rate, which compares the number of deaths with the whole population, not just those with the disease. The case fatality rate gives an idea of how deadly a disease is – for example, rabies in an unvaccinated and untreated person has a case fatality rate of almost 100%.

How long patients survive following a diagnosis or a treatment can be calculated as a survival rate as already described, but another way is to consider the *median survival. This refers to the time when half the patients are expected to be alive.* Again this does not refer to individuals; some may live much longer and others much shorter than the median. There will always be outliers where survival times are very different to the average; this is why median is used rather than mean survival. This would be helpful for a clinical commissioning group trying to work out the typical length of service provision needed for a group of patients (*see* Question 6.2).

Kaplan–Meier curves give a graphical presentation of the survival rates following diagnosis or treatment. Often incomplete data are held about a disease or treatment and Kaplan–Meier estimates are used to complete the data. This is most commonly presented as a survival curve (although Kaplan–Meier estimates can be used for other expected events, not just survival). The curve can be based on overall survival of other estimates, such as disease-free survival or progression-free survival. Sometimes the estimates are of disease-specific survival and not all-cause mortality. Make sure you look at exactly what is being presented.

Q 6.16 Meningitis from meningococcal disease has a peak incidence in children under 1 year old. It is responsible for more deaths of children under 5 in the UK than any other infectious disease. In 2011/12 there were 764 new cases of invasive meningococcal disease in England and Wales across all ages. The population of England and Wales was about 54.5 million. What was the incidence of invasive meningococcal disease across all ages in those 12 months? Give the rate per 100 000 people. Write your answer in the box provided.

Q 6.17 The number of deaths from the 764 new cases of invasive meningococcal disease over the 12 months of 2011/12 was 38. What was the case fatality rate? Write your answer in the box provided.

The information given in Question 6.16 about meningitis tells us that there were 764 new cases in a population of 54.5 million. To make the calculation of incidence easier and to give us a rate per 100 000, first divide 54.5 million by 100 000: this gives us 545. Then divide the number of cases of meningococcal disease by 545 to give a rate per 100 000.

$$\frac{764}{545} = 1.4 \text{ per } 100\,000$$

To work out the case fatality rate you divide the number of deaths by the total number of people who had the disease. In this case there were 38 deaths in 764 cases.

$$\frac{38}{764} = 0.0497 = 5\%$$

Therefore the case fatality rate was just under 5%, or almost one in 20 cases of invasive meningococcal disease resulted in death. A quarter of the deaths were in children younger than 1 year old. This disease also causes significant morbidity.

ECONOMIC AND QUALITY OF LIFE ANALYSIS

Modern medical and surgical care is very expensive. In many countries the cost of health systems is a large proportion of total government expenditure. In countries where healthcare is funded through an insurance model, the cost is similarly very high. Because of this, it is important to know whether new (or existing) treatments can be considered to be economically viable in relation to the expected improvement in health they may bring. If a treatment is able to offer a cure for a disease, it may be very cost-effective because the cost of caring for people with that disease will be avoided. However, if a treatment provides a small benefit for a large number of people, it may be equally cost-effective by reducing the future care needs of those people.

There are several ways of considering whether a treatment is cost-effective. First of all the treatment needs to be adequately assessed for effectiveness; the treatment has to be shown to work and an idea of how effective it is and in which group of people needs to be understood. Once the effectiveness of a treatment is known, it can then be related to the cost of that treatment. Obviously, a cheap treatment that is highly effective is great for healthcare, but an expensive treatment that has limited effectiveness needs to be considered against how willing people (or governments, or insurers) are to pay for it.

This is where measures such as *QALYs, or quality-adjusted life years*, are helpful. *A QALY is a standardised measure for comparing different treatments*. It is the *average number of **additional** years of life gained from a treatment multiplied by a factor that takes into account the quality of life* that may be expected in those additional years of life. This needs a relatively objective way of considering quality of life; this is sometimes gained by conducting interviews and questionnaires with people with the condition of interest and receiving the treatment(s) of interest.

One QALY is a year of life gained with 'perfect' health. The closer to 1 the quality of life is taken to be, the better it is (a score of 1 being healthy quality of life). It is possible to have a negative quality of life, where living for additional years could be considered worse than allowing a patient to die.

QALYs can be difficult to interpret and there can be debate about how valid the quality of life calculation is. They are calculated by taking the expected life expectancy of a person and considering how many years of additional life may be expected by having a treatment.

An example of calculating a QALY is as follows: a person is expected to live 10 years longer if on blood pressure-reducing medication, which the person takes for 20 years before he or she dies. This is compared with the change in his or her quality of life for those 20 years. The person's quality of life will be reduced through having to take the tablets and through any side effects that he or she experiences, as well as through being older and frailer.

This gives an **additional** 10 years of life at a slightly reduced quality of life compared with that previously experienced. If the quality of life of those additional 10 years is taken to be 0.9, this gives a loss of quality of life of 0.1 per year. The 20 years of taking medication slightly reduces quality of life also – this may be quantified as a loss of quality of life of 0.02 per year.

The full calculation in this example would be the additional years gained minus the quality of life lost during those 10 years and the quality of life lost throughout the 20 years of taking tablets.

$$10 - (10 \times 0.1) - (20 \times 0.02) = 10 - 1 - 0.4 = 8.6 \text{ years}$$

This means that the additional 10 years of life would be equivalent to 8.6 extra years of life. The higher the QALY, the better the treatment is.

DALYs, or disability-adjusted life years, take the **negative** *impact of disability into account. One DALY represents 1 lost year of healthy life.* DALYs consider how much disability or disease reduces life expectancy, by comparing the life spans of people with the disease to that of the overall population. They also consider how much the impact of the disease affects quality of life. This is done in a similar way to calculating a QALY. Someone with a serious disease that is diagnosed at the age of 70 may have been expected to live to 80 but dies aged 72 – losing 8 years of life expectancy. The quality of those 2 years between diagnosis and death may be considered to be worth only 1 year of healthy life, so another year of healthy life is lost. Therefore, in this case, the calculation would give a DALY of 9 years of healthy life lost.

The role of DALYs is in comparing the impact of disease and also allowing health professionals to concentrate finite resources on those diseases that cause the highest loss of healthy life. This is done by comparing the DALYs for a population. For example, if road traffic collisions are causing a greater loss of life and a large increase in disability, this may be a priority for public health interventions leading to such measures as making seatbelts compulsory in motor vehicles.

Cost-benefit analysis uses a large variety of techniques, including looking at QALYs and DALYs in comparison with the cost of treatments. The most cost-effective treatment is calculated in several ways but it is essentially looking for the treatment that has the best effect for the lowest cost. If a treatment has a good outcome but is very expensive, it may not be possible to fund that treatment in a public healthcare system, because it will mean other, more cost-effective treatments cannot be funded. The National Institute for Health and Care Excellence in the UK uses a cost per QALY calculation to decide whether treatments are cost-effective. The threshold for considering a drug cost-effective is currently between £20 000 and £30 000 per QALY gained.

The main problems with cost-benefit analyses are how to measure and assign a value to different costs and benefits. Some things are easy to measure, such as the cost of a drug, but there are often things, such as improved or worsened symptoms, that are difficult to assign a value to. Also bear in mind that different healthcare organisations ascribe different costs and benefits to the same treatments.

CHAPTER 7

Research in general practice

INTRODUCTION

As GPs we need to view our patients as individuals. Sometimes we face complex clinical scenarios where following guidance may be inappropriate. If a patient has a flare of his or her rheumatoid arthritis and is already taking warfarin, digoxin and furosemide, it may not be appropriate to treat that patient with steroids or non-steroidal anti-inflammatory drugs (NSAIDs). We are responsible for coordinating the care of our patients and sometimes there will be conflicting advice from different specialists. We have to take an overall view of the patient and incorporate his or her preferences and concerns into decision-making.

We need to be able to help patients decide on the best treatment options, no matter how complex their health needs or medical history. In order to do this, we need to be able to formulate clinical questions and know how to find the answers. There are several ways of doing this. Realistically, there is not a great deal of time to find answers to clinical questions within a consultation or within the working week, so we need several strategies to find and use good evidence. One option is to refer to national guidance.

Guidance should be based on the best available evidence, so it can be very useful in deciding on treatment options for patients. However, sometimes the guidance available does not cover the complexity of patients we see. When we decide that we cannot follow guidance, we are often at the limits of our knowledge or even at the limits of evidence-based practice. It may be that the best evidence cannot inform us of the best course of action for an individual patient. This is a criticism of evidence-based medicine that is often raised, in that it looks at medicine at a population level rather than the level of the individual consulting his or her doctor. There are other limits to evidence-based medicine that we should be aware of and these will be discussed briefly in Chapter 8.

Before we reach a discussion of the limits of evidence-based medicine, we need to focus on how to practise it. We need to know how to formulate and answer clinical questions that are aimed at improving the care of our patients. When guidance cannot answer our clinical questions, we need to ask the right questions and know where to look for the answers. This chapter is primarily focused on the UK but most of the resources mentioned here will be useful for primary care internationally.

There are two strands to research in primary care. The first is that already introduced, knowing how to ask and answer clinical questions that arise in our consultations with patients. The other strand is research programmes that are based in general practice. Many practices will be involved in research projects that are either endeavouring to discover how best to treat patients in general practice or looking at longer-term outcomes for patients on particular medications or particular conditions.

Every practice should also monitor outcomes for its own patients. This is often done through audits but can also be undertaken using significant event analysis (a case study). A lot of the knowledge GPs have is informally shared; often our first port of call when we have a question is to ask our colleagues if they know a reasonable answer. This is quicker and is a more effective use of time when there are so many other things that need to be done.

However, colleagues may not always be able to answer our questions, and on occasion they may base their answer on old, possibly superseded or incorrectly remembered knowledge. This is when we have to turn to other sources. There are a lot of organisations now devoted to improving the evidence base for medicine and there are also organisations that aim to disseminate this information.

Q 7.1   For what purpose would you use PICO?
a) Analysing data for a systematic review
b) Considering whether a randomised controlled trial gives an accurate result
c) Formulating a question for a research topic
d) Formulating a question for a search strategy
e) Considering the appropriateness of a statistical test

Q 7.2   What does PICO stand for? More than one answer may be correct.
a) Pretty indicative controlled outcome
b) Problem, intervention, control, outcome
c) Problem, intention, context, outcome
d) Priority, intervention, comparison, outcome
e) Population, intervention, comparison, outcome

Q 7.3   Put the following steps in the correct order for an audit cycle.
a) Select appropriate criteria and set standards.
b) Repeat the audit.
c) Select a topic.
d) Identify areas for improvement and setting actions to achieve improvement.
e) Collect data and measure performance.

Q 7.4   From the following options, choose the best definition for 'optimum standard'.
a) The standard of care most likely under normal conditions
b) The best possible standard of care
c) The minimum acceptable standard of care
d) The standard of care that will avoid any harm to patients
e) The average standard of care

AUDIT

You should have undertaken audits during your training. Audits are a way of assessing and evaluating the care of our patients and they provide a way of identifying areas of our care that should be improved. Audits should be repeated at appropriate intervals to ensure that appropriate care for our patients is maintained. Undertaking audits is a requirement of the General Medical Council in the UK, in order that doctors maintain and improve their practice. It is also a requirement of revalidation; it is expected that in a 5-year revalidation cycle you will complete an audit cycle.

The audit cycle includes several steps. First, a topic needs to be selected, preferably one that is a priority for you or your organisation. The selection of a topic often arises from clinical need or through learning of appropriate care standards as part of continuing professional development.

The second step is to select appropriate criteria and a standard that you will audit against. The criteria often take the form of an idealised statement, such as 'all patients with increased cardiovascular disease risk should have their blood pressure monitored at least once a year'. The standard may be a minimum that would be acceptable, it may be an ideal or it may lie somewhere between the two. The optimum standard represents the standard of care most likely under normal conditions. The criteria and standards should be based on the best available evidence and are often based on guidelines.

The third step in an audit cycle is to collect the data and analyse it. You compare the data collected with the standards already chosen. This is an opportunity to think about why standards were or were not met.

The crucial fourth step is identifying areas for improvement and discussing these with colleagues, in order that improvements can be made by the whole organisation. It is essential that any action needed is clearly set out and individuals know what is expected of them. Setting a time frame is also important.

Finally, the audit should be repeated at an appropriate interval to make sure that the actions taken have been effective and have led to the expected improvements in care. This may go on for several cycles or it may be accepted that the ideal level of care has been met and so the audit cycle could be considered completed.

HOW TO ANSWER QUESTIONS RELEVANT TO PRIMARY CARE

When you have a patient in front of you who has a particular disease, such as rheumatoid arthritis, you may have several questions about his or her treatment. The patient may have other medical conditions such as hypertension, heart failure or renal impairment. You may be interested in whether the patient should be on a statin or whether this may make his or her symptoms worse or put him or her at risk of developing diabetes. You may want to know whether treating the patient's arthritis with an NSAID will put him or her at greater risk of a heart attack, and if so, you may want to be able to quantify the risk so that the patient can make an informed choice about treatment.

Being able to formulate a question about the clinical care of a patient and knowing how to answer that question can provide better care for that patient. A basic question may need further clarification in order to find helpful, specific information quickly. One way that has been suggested for formulating questions is the PICO framework. Here the P stands for patient, population or problem; I stands for intervention or exposure (to a drug or risk factor); C stands for comparison or control; and O stands for outcome.

The initial question may be: 'Is it appropriate to use an NSAID for someone with arthritis and ischaemic heart disease?' This question formulated using the PICO framework would be: *'In patients with rheumatoid arthritis and heart disease (P), by how much does the use of an NSAID (I) compared with the use of simple analgesia (C) increase the risk of myocardial infarction (O)?'* This helps you judge which information is useful in the clinical scenario you face and also means you can use more focused search terms to discover helpful answers quickly. Most of the evidence-based medicine resources will have advanced search facilities so that you can include all the relevant terms you need.

Once you have some results, you will want to evaluate these for how useful they are in answering your question. The most helpful evidence may be from meta-analyses or systematic reviews, followed by that from good-quality randomised controlled trials. Sometimes the only available evidence is that of expert opinion. You will have to evaluate the findings for yourself, and this includes not only looking for the appropriateness of the evidence but also looking at the methods to assess for possible sources of bias and weaknesses. Often the methods expose the limitations of the study and will allow you to decide whether this research can be applied to your patient.

However, there are some problems with this method. It is time-consuming, and even when you appear to have an answer, you will need to evaluate the evidence it is based upon. This may call on skills that are rusty and may involve more time than is practical when you have many other patients to see and treat. Also evidence is often contingent – there is often a need for further studies to clarify evidence, which means you would have to repeat your search periodically to remain up to date.

Fortunately, there are ways around these problems. There are resources that do the searching, summarising and evaluating for you or with you. These resources include journal clubs, synopses and review databases. Often these are the best places to start a search. There are also resources that allow you to ask your question and then a specialist will look for and summarise the results. Librarians in hospital libraries are frequently able to do this for you. Disseminating the information you find to your colleagues is very helpful, because it can save other clinicians a great deal of time and can help keep knowledge up to date.

EVIDENCE-BASED RESOURCES

There are many evidence-based resources available. Most of these are located on the Internet. Here we introduce a few of them, but undoubtedly you will have other resources that you use. First, though, it is worth thinking about how to evaluate resources and how to get the most helpful information from them. If they are to be helpful, it is important that these resources are based on the best available evidence and that they are kept up to date.

When looking at a resource you should ask yourself several basic questions. Who is behind the resource? Are they a reputable organisation without obvious biases? Where does the funding for the resource come from? Does the funding organisation have any input into the way evidence is presented and discussed? Is the evidence reviewed and up to date? Is the evidence presented in a clear, accessible way with some indication of revision when necessary? Are the methods used for evaluating evidence transparent and appropriate?

If a resource is easy to search and use, then you are more likely to use it when pressed for time. It also needs to have reliable evidence presented in a clear way. This means that methods used to evaluate evidence should be published and easy to locate. Even very helpful and trusted websites may not meet all these criteria, but if you are aware of any shortcomings, you can take these into account when using these resources.

RESEARCH DATABASES AND NETWORKS

There are a great number of research databases and evidence-based medicine resources. We will look at only a few. These are UK-based resources but there are similar resources in many other countries.

The **National Institute for Health and Care Excellence**, or NICE (www.nice.org.uk), is the national organisation in the UK that produces guidance and advice aimed at improving health and social care. These guidelines are based on appraising the evidence for both clinical and cost-effectiveness. NICE is independent of government and its guidelines are made by independent committees. The work of NICE has, it can be argued, transformed the way clinicians work in the UK and is very much at the forefront of implementing evidence-based practice. Guidelines are only for guidance, they do not have to be followed; however, if they are not followed, it is wise to have clear reasons for not doing so. When faced with a patient with multiple chronic diseases, it may not be appropriate to follow guidance; rather, it may be appropriate to develop a strategy for investigation and management with the patient. The reason for this is that guidance is normally focused on one disease and cannot take full account of the complexity of individual presentations.

NICE also provides **NICE Evidence** (www.evidence.nhs.uk), which is a search engine for clinical, public health and social care guidance. This web-based service also includes Clinical Knowledge Summaries, UK DUETs and evidence awareness services. The search engine covers a wide range of sources of information including international and national journals, medical colleges and associations and third sector organisations' websites.

Clinical Knowledge Summaries (http://cks.nice.org.uk) are useful summaries of current evidence and they offer practical guidance on how to treat selected conditions. There is a broad range of conditions included in Clinical Knowledge Summaries, although they do not have comprehensive coverage of all clinical conditions. The main advantage of Clinical Knowledge Summaries is that they are very quick to digest and they set out treatment options clearly. They are updated regularly, although there is obviously a lag between new evidence emerging and it being incorporated.

UK DUETs (www.library.nhs.uk/duets/) is a database of uncertainties about the effects of treatments. This draws on patients' and clinicians' experiences and questions about the effects of treatments. It also draws on research recommendations in systematic reviews and guidelines. The database includes a brief explanation of why there is uncertainty and suggestions of what needs to be done to tackle these uncertainties – for example, it may be that systematic reviews are out of date and need updating. When using the best evidence, we should admit to patients that there are areas of uncertainty even around quite established treatments; this is a fundamental part of evidence-based practice. There are always benefits, costs and uncertainties of treatment and patients have a right to know what these are, as fully as clinicians do.

The Cochrane Library (www.thecochranelibrary.com) is based on the work of Archie Cochrane who, in the 1970s, drew attention to the lack of knowledge about the effects of healthcare. He suggested that systematic reviews of evidence should be performed and updated regularly. The Cochrane Library now includes several databases. The most well-known is the Cochrane Database of Systematic Reviews, but there is also the Cochrane Central Register of Controlled Trials, the Health Technology Assessment Database, the Database of Abstracts of Reviews of Effects, and the National Health Service (NHS) Economic Evaluation Database. These last three databases are produced by the Centre for Reviews and Dissemination at the University of York. The Database of Abstracts of Reviews of Effects gives an abstract of systematic reviews along with an assessment of the overall quality of the systematic review. The NHS Economic Evaluation Database and the Health Technology Assessment Database include cost-effectiveness studies from around the world to enable decisions to be made regarding the implementation of healthcare interventions.

A very interesting collaboration between clinicians, researchers and patients is the **James Lind Alliance** (www.lindalliance.org). The aim of this organisation is to include patients in setting research priorities. They hold workshops with patients, clinicians and others to find out where there are uncertainties about treatments but moreover to prioritise research based on what the patients themselves want to know. This is incredibly useful for researchers setting out on research projects and helping them maintain a focus on the people who will actually benefit from or be harmed by treatments. In a similar way to UK DUETs, this work sets out quite clearly that there are a lot of uncertainties about the treatments we use or may be considering using and patients need to be aware of these.

The **Trip database** (www.tripdatabase.com) is a search engine with the aim of allowing users to quickly and easily find high-quality research evidence. Trip allows you to do a basic search, an advanced search or a search with PICO terms. This links through to sources such as PubMed or the Centre for Reviews and Dissemination to allow you to read the abstracts of relevant articles. You can refine your results by evidence type, such as systematic reviews or guidelines. Results can be refined in other ways such as images or patient information. This has an advantage over general search engines in that it only looks for evidence from appropriate resources.

These are just a few of the resources available. There are other organisations producing helpful evidence-based resources, such as the BMJ Evidence Centre from the BMJ Group (http://group.bmj.com/products/evidence-centre). Finding a resource that works for you is the most important factor in enabling you to use evidence-based resources.

RESEARCH IN GENERAL PRACTICE

As a GP, you can become involved in research if you have questions that you would like answered and for which there is not a clear answer in the literature. Being involved in research helps GPs stay up to date and can offer opportunities to improve the care of your patients. There is also personal satisfaction in undertaking research that helps improve the care of our patients.

A very simple way of becoming involved in research is by gaining patient consent for data to be uploaded to a central data hub. Data from general practice can be used to investigate many clinical problems. There is a huge amount of data collected in general practice. Each consultation is recorded along with clinical codes for problems and diagnoses and lists of medication, all of which can form the basis for research. This was recognised when computerised record keeping became more commonplace in the 1980s in the UK. The **General Practice Research Database** was founded in 1987 to collect primary care data. This collected data from all four countries of the UK and covered about 8% of the UK population.

As GPs, we occupy a central role in the NHS whereby we act as both provider of primary care and referrer to secondary care. Nearly all information regarding our patients' medical treatment will come to us. Even if patients choose to access private healthcare, letters will be sent back to their GP. When patients move practice, their records follow them and so there should be a continuous record of healthcare for individuals. This gives a wealth of longitudinal data. This data relies on GP practices accurately coding the information they receive about patients. The information they add to the record must also be coded to allow the database to search for that information.

Anonymised data from general practices is collected by the **Clinical Practice Research Datalink** (www.cprd.com) in the UK (this has grown from and incorporates the General Practice Research Database). It is funded by the NHS National Institute for Health Research and the Medicines and Healthcare Products Regulatory Agency (MHRA). This database has been used in hundreds of studies. Links with other countries have been developed in order to increase the data set and provide research that can compare outcomes in different countries. Coverage of the UK population is also being expanded so that the database becomes more comprehensive and therefore more useful. Data is anonymised before researchers can use it so that individual patients are not identifiable from the data provided. There are similar databases in other countries.

The *National Institute for Health Research Primary Care Research Network* aims to provide researchers with practical support to undertake clinical studies in primary care in England. Primary care includes doctors, nurses, dentists, pharmacists, opticians, care homes, health visitors and anyone else involved with primary care. The aim is to help improve treatments for patients and also to target NHS resources where they will be most effective. They help both GPs and patients become involved in research. Training for GPs is provided to enable them to participate in research projects.

Normally the research projects are undertaken by academic or commercial organisations. The primary care research network ensures that clinical studies are of high quality and supports researchers and GP practices in undertaking the research. GP practices decide which studies they wish to become involved with and the commitment necessary ranges from a clinical record search through to having patients start randomised treatments when they present with particular symptoms. Trials and studies undertaken in primary care are always in need of participants.

There are similar networks in Scotland (the Scottish Primary Care Research Network), Northern Ireland (the Northern Ireland Clinical Research Network) and Wales (the National Institute for Social Care and Health Research Clinical Research Centre) as well as a wider European network (the European General Practice Research Network). These all provide some level of support to GPs involved in research and also provide a forum to discuss research opportunities and problems.

The Royal College of General Practitioners encourages research through its **Clinical Innovation and Research Centre**. The aim is to provide research leadership by identifying priorities for research, securing funding and disseminating research findings. The Royal College of General Practitioners also has a research and surveillance centre that monitors infection rates for communicable diseases, particularly flu.

SOCIAL NETWORKING

As well as the more formal research networks already mentioned, there are thriving communities based on social media. These can be excellent ways of finding research projects, accessing support and asking questions when considering starting research in general practice. There are often people willing to engage with you when you have a question. This is very like asking your colleagues their opinion about something but with a much wider reach and potentially a much wider spread of opinion. Researchers often post links to interesting studies. As with any community, you have to be wary of incorrect information and misleading information. The benefits outweigh potential disadvantages if you remember to use the same level of scepticism that you would with any other form of knowledge transfer.

RESEARCH ETHICS

Research ethics are the principles that researchers should keep to in order to maintain trust, integrity, objectivity, confidentiality, competence and honesty in research. There are various codes that address research ethics. The **Declaration of Helsinki**, originally adopted by the World Medical Association in 1964, is widely regarded as the most important of these in medicine. This has undergone several revisions and clarifications since then, the latest of which was in 2013. The fundamental principle in the Declaration is that the first consideration of a researcher should be the health of his or her patient and all actions will be in the best interests of his or her patients. The rights of the individual always take precedence over other interests.

Good Clinical Practice is an international set of standards for quality in research involving human subjects. To some degree this has become more important than the Declaration of Helsinki for clinical researchers. The aim is to ensure that trials protect human rights and ensure the collection of good-quality data. The European Union published a **Clinical Trials Directive** in 2001, which was revised in 2013 and has similar aims.

All medical research in the UK (and most other countries) undertaken with human participants, tissue samples or data has to be approved by an independent research ethics committee. This is to protect research participants' privacy and to ensure that research is undertaken appropriately, with safeguards to ensure the risk of harm is minimised. The NHS uses independent ethics committees that are part of the Health Research Authority's National Research Ethics Service.

Before a research project can start, a detailed plan needs to be submitted to a research ethics committee setting out how the research is to be conducted. These committees have to include members who are not health professionals. Clinical trials are subject to legal obligations set out in the Medicines for Human Uses (Clinical Trials) Regulations 2004. The MHRA has to authorise all clinical trials of medicines. The MHRA also inspects research sites to make sure trials are conducted in line with good clinical practice standards.

Researchers should prepare a patient information leaflet or pack. Participants should be able to make an informed choice about taking part in the research and understand that they can withdraw at any time. The information participants should be provided with includes the research questions that the research is aiming to answer; who can and who cannot take part in the trial; what is expected of participants; potential risks and benefits; who is funding the trial and who participants should contact if they have any questions or concerns. Only once a trial has research ethics approval can researchers start recruiting participants and collecting data. The consent of participants should be clearly recorded. Of course, confidentiality has to be maintained throughout the research process.

Maintaining an ethical stance does not finish once the trial data are collected and analysed. If not all trial data are published, this can alter the apparent efficacy of medications. It is important that all trials are published and all data are available to researchers to study and incorporate into meta-analyses. This is the aim of the campaign AllTrials (www.alltrials.net), to have all clinical trials registered and all results reported. You will remember that in Chapter 5 we saw how funnel plots can show if there is significant publication bias. We need complete evidence where possible, in order to make the best decisions regarding patient care, to avoid harm to our patients and to enable informed decision-making.

Unfortunately, research fraud occurs all too frequently and in many guises. This ranges from fabricating data to researchers peer-reviewing papers in which they have been involved. Every year there are many papers that are retracted. Some of these retractions are because of research fraud while others are because of mistakes in interpreting data. If researchers do not act in line with research ethics, the damage to the medical profession can be profound. Research that found a link between the MMR vaccine and autism is an example of this. The papers in which this claim was made have been retracted and most of the authors of those papers have issued corrections stating no link was found between MMR and autism. Despite all of this, there are still people who refuse to let their children have the MMR vaccine because of fears of autism.

DISCUSSING TREATMENTS WITH PATIENTS

Once research has been completed and published it has to be put into use. GPs need ways of helping patients to make decisions about possible treatment options. Uncertainties constantly arise in medicine. A skilled doctor needs to communicate those uncertainties in a way appropriate to each individual patient. Risk is uncertainty about future events represented as a probability; this should be based on research findings, so being aware of the evidence is vital. The level of risk that patients are willing to accept varies enormously and that is why they should be involved in decision-making.

The NHS has a website, Shared Decision Making, devoted to patient decision aids that people can use to come to the best decision for them (http://sdm.rightcare.nhs.uk). Each decision aid provides information on available options and allows patients to consider what is important to them in coming to a decision. These decision aids can be used before or following an initial consultation, allowing patients time to weigh up their options.

For some people, presenting data visually can be more helpful than written information. One way of doing this is with a Cates plot (www.nntonline.net). A Cates plot employs 'smiley faces' in red, yellow and green. A chart of 100 or 1000 smiley faces is presented. People who would have a good outcome are shown as green smiley faces, whereas people who would have a bad outcome are shown as red frowning faces. Yellow faces are used for people in whom treatment changes a bad outcome to a good outcome. Crossed out green faces are used to represent treatment causing an adverse outcome. There are other similar charts that use different icons.

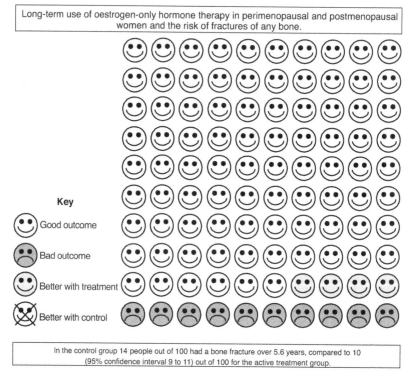

FIGURE 7.1 A Cates plot showing the risk of fracture for women taking oestrogen-only hormone replacement therapy over 5.6 years[*]

These plots are based on odds ratios or relative risk published in systematic reviews, and they calculate the number needed to treat. As you will remember

---

[*] Created using data from table 6.27 in Marjoribanks J, Farquhar C, Roberts H, *et al.* Long term hormone therapy for perimenopausal and postmenopausal women. *Cochrane Database Syst Rev.* 2012; 7: CD004143. Created using the web-based free software Visual Rx at www.nntonline.net

from Chapter 5, these figures change depending on the timescale used, so this should be considered when interpreting these plots. The plot shown in Figure 7.1, for example, is based on treatment with oestrogen-only hormone replacement therapy for 5.6 years. Also remember that these plots are based on the pooled data from meta-analyses or other studies; you cannot determine which category a patient will fall into.

APPLYING STATISTICS TO INDIVIDUALS

Several times in the preceding chapters we have mentioned the difficulties inherent in applying statistics to individuals. We know that some statistical methods can be directly applied to individuals but we also know that many statistical outcomes apply only to a population. This is an often-cited criticism of evidence-based medicine – that as physicians we treat individuals but evidence is largely about groups of people. This is called an ecological fallacy, when attributes of an individual are deduced from the attributes of the group to which the individual belongs. It is clear that the attributes of an individual within a group will vary from the average of that group. Correlations between variables for a group will not necessarily translate into correlations that apply to individuals.

What does this mean for us as GPs? We treat individuals but within a resource-limited system; we need to be aware of the impact of our decisions for individuals on the wider population. We cannot afford to treat one patient with an intervention that costs so much that many other individuals would not be able to benefit from other cheap and effective interventions. This is where our clinical judgement has to be tempered by our knowledge of the opportunity cost of our decisions. This is also where the knowledge of public health professionals can be very helpful.

Some of the problems with evidence-based medicine are discussed in the next chapter. We will also look at what comes next for evidence-based medicine.

CHAPTER 8

Conclusions

INTRODUCTION

After reading through this book and practising the questions, you should have a good understanding of how research works, how to evaluate research and how to calculate some important statistics. This book is not a comprehensive introduction to statistics, research methods or even evidence-based practice; rather, its aim is to get you through the AKT and, it is to be hoped, to inspire you to become an evidence-based practitioner. Being able to appropriately use evidence and knowing when to look for evidence are two fundamental skills for GPs. If you can use evidence in conjunction with good communication, you will be able to provide better care to your patients.

Just as other areas of enquiry are forged within paradigms (the prevailing practices and culture of an area of study), this is also true of statistics. The dominant paradigm in biostatistics as taught to doctors is the frequentist one. The frequentist approach uses the hypothesis testing model that results in a confidence interval around what is assumed to be a fixed value. Most of the content of this book is based upon that paradigm, but there are challenges based on other approaches – particularly Bayesian methods. Bayesian methods allow for unknown values to have a probability distribution rather than a fixed value.

Combining pre-test odds with the likelihood ratio to estimate post-test odds, as we did in Chapter 6, employs a Bayesian approach. We can use this Bayesian approach in clinical decision-making. The pre-test probability may be the clinician's impression of the disease prevalence. The likelihood ratio is represented by the strength of evidence gained from symptoms, signs or investigations. The product of the pre-test probability and likelihood ratio gives the post-test probability of the patient having the disease. In practice we often do this without thinking about numbers or statistics; we weigh up the chance of a patient having a particular disease based on our knowledge of the patient and what is common or rare.

We do not expect you to be overly interested in these debates about paradigms and varying approaches but you should be aware that changes in medical knowledge over time are mirrored in biostatistics – it is not a static area of knowledge but one that changes, with new ideas and techniques being constantly developed.

In this chapter, we look at challenges for evidence-based medicine and possible influences on the way that medicine will be practised over the coming decades. There will always be a place for generalists with a talent for identifying what is important for their patients and who are able to communicate with their patients in ways that enable better understanding and better care. Before we look at these challenges, though, it is worth recapping the fundamentals of how to succeed in the AKT.

HOW TO SUCCEED IN THE APPLIED KNOWLEDGE TEST

This book is about only one strand of the AKT. Knowing that you can score highly on the questions about research and statistics will boost your overall chance of success in the exam. There are no secrets to doing well – you simply need to put in the appropriate work. By reading this book you have increased your chances of successfully passing the AKT. Make sure that you have practised the questions in Chapters 2–7 and Chapter 9. Make sure you understand why the answer is correct. If you have difficulty with any particular area, go back to the relevant section of the book and reread it and then practise the questions again. If you are still struggling, then make up your own questions with simple figures and work out the correct answers using the information in the text. Being able to explain why you have arrived at the answer you know to be correct will be the sign that you truly understand what you are doing.

Reread the suggestions in Chapter 1 as to how to prepare for the AKT and make sure you start to prepare in plenty of time. Consider how you learn best and utilise the methods that work best for you. If you are struggling with something, take time to speak to colleagues and get answers to your questions. Focus on and put more effort into those areas that you know you struggle with until you feel comfortable with any questions relevant to them. Finally, try to put into practice what you have learnt. The best way of remembering something is to apply it in real life.

WHAT NEXT? HOW IS EVIDENCE-BASED MEDICINE DEVELOPING?

Throughout this book there have been hints of some of the problems that evidence-based medicine faces. At the end of the previous chapter we talked about the ecological fallacy – the problem of applying statistical results based on the study of groups to individuals. Does this matter? To some extent this depends on what the underpinning philosophy of evidence-based medicine is taken to be. If you rigorously apply statistical methods and interpret the results carefully, you will draw more circumscribed conclusions that may be less applicable to other situations. If you have a more relaxed approach to applying statistical methods and to interpreting the results, you may draw much more widely applicable conclusions. The problem is drawing valid conclusions. The former approach may be falsely limiting and the latter approach may go far beyond what is appropriate. An important point is that evidence-based medicine may be incredibly powerful and helpful in improving patient outcomes but it is only one aspect of improving medicine and its techniques need to be applied appropriately.

This chapter is different from the others in this book: it will not directly help you to pass the AKT – in fact, it will not necessarily be of any interest to you at this stage in your career. However, it is included here as an acknowledgement that there are limits to evidence-based medicine and that medical practice is constantly changing. It is a provocation to think more deeply about the underpinnings of evidence-based practice and an invitation to consider future medical practice. After all, you may have several decades of medical practice ahead of you and these issues will be of importance to you in future if you are to remain an honest and reflective practitioner.

As evidence-based medicine is widely accepted – it is taught in most medical schools after all – it follows that there are more people drawing more conclusions from the evidence that we have. There are attempts to standardise the way conclusions are drawn but these are not without their problems. The Cochrane systematic reviews have been criticised for taking too much resource to complete and they take a lot of time to complete so the final number of reviews is limited. The argument follows that usable evidence can be produced through quicker but more limited systematic reviews.

Evidence-based medicine practitioners accept that some of our current practice, taken as accepted based on the available evidence, will turn out to be incorrect. This is the nature of the improvement of our knowledge. There will be false turns and dead ends. There will also undoubtedly be harm to our patients, both because the evidence is not appreciated and because the evidence is applied incorrectly.

As knowledge improves, so it is to be hoped will our treatment of our patients. However, it is recognised that even when evidence is clear, it takes many years before the majority of clinicians are applying that evidence with their patients. The reasons for this are complex, but it may be because evidence is not translated quickly enough into useable information that is easily understood and applied by busy clinicians. It may also be because clinicians are more comfortable sticking with the interventions they have seen to work with previous patients. It may also be because clinicians are aware of the limits of evidence and recognise that conclusions change as more research is conducted.

We need more than just quantitative methodology if we are to understand and improve the care of our patients. We need to develop qualitative understanding of our patients' experiences. This is especially true for GPs, particularly given that we deal with much that may not be considered to be 'medical' within a narrow definition of that term. Dealing with family breakdown, suicidal feelings and job-related stress will not be helped by statistical analysis as much as it will be helped by understanding the experiences of our patients.

Evidence-based medicine prioritises that which can be quantitatively described, and some things will not fit into that pattern. In many fields of the humanities and social sciences there was a twentieth-century movement labelled 'logical positivism' that did something similar in bringing quantitative analysis to the forefront of those fields. Interestingly, these academic disciplines have rejected or greatly modified logical positivism for more complex understandings of how the world works. Evidence-based medicine may have to reconsider its hierarchy of evidence and accept that other types of evidence can also be helpful, particularly when dealing with individuals.

Other problems with the hierarchy of evidence are debated. For example, there is an argument that randomised controlled trials are not the gold standard they are often taken to be. There is an argument that RCTs are open to several types of bias and even double-blind controlled trials will not eliminate these biases. It is also argued that randomised selection cannot eliminate differences occurring between control and experimental arms. More important, RCTs do not always investigate those people who will be the likely recipients of the interventions of interest. Although all of these arguments can be countered, the more fundamental problem with the hierarchy of evidence is that there are many powerful and clinically useful studies that are not RCTs and some evidence simply cannot be formed through RCTs. The hierarchy of evidence has to be understood to be an idealised system that has many contradictions and flaws in practice.

Another fundamental problem for evidence-based medicine is that research often neglects practice. What does this mean? Research often does not take into account current clinical practice or what could possibly become accepted clinical practice. We have all seen RCTs that test against placebo rather than against the current accepted best practice. Moreover, RCTs often do not have outcomes that can be easily applied to clinical practice. Remember that any statistic is an answer to a specific question, correlation does not mean causation and the questions being asked have to be refined for research to be worthwhile.

There is a failure to translate research into practice. This is a big challenge for evidence-based medicine. Without translating research into practice, there is no point in completing the research. It is important to acknowledge that some research needs to be conducted on basic mechanisms that will not be translatable to practice. However, it is arguable that there is not the right balance between this category of research and research that will have an impact on patient treatments.

There are growing volumes of guidelines and evidence. No busy doctor or healthcare professional could reasonably be expected to know all the latest evidence and guidelines, nor could he or she be expected to adhere to them. Real life is often more complex than that presented in guidelines. GPs have conceivably the toughest task in keeping up with evidence of any doctors, because they are expected to know about such a wide, and increasing, range of conditions. In the UK, GPs are also taking on more and more of the work that used to be done in hospitals. Do we need a fundamental rethink on how GPs are expected to work?

Another problem with guidelines is that there are often international, national and local guidelines and some of these inevitably conflict. Which should be followed? Even more challenging is the funding of medicine – guidelines can increase direct and indirect costs. Even when treatments are deemed more cost-effective than existing practice, there is the cost of changing practice – if hospital departments are set up to follow previous guidelines and these change, there can be a huge cost in terms of training and equipment. Furthermore, guidelines may increase both financial and health costs by making professionals more risk averse (if guidelines are not followed, it is more likely that a professional will be vilified or sanctioned) and therefore more likely to investigate those who previously may have benefited from a watchful waiting approach.

Evidence-based medicine is incredibly helpful and has overseen a very positive revolution in medical practice. The criticisms levelled here are not to disparage that impact but are an acceptance that paradigms change and evidence-based practice will also change.

It feels as if evidence-based medicine has only just been accepted into mainstream medical practice (though this has actually been happening for about 20 or 30 years, or even longer if you take into account the work of Archie Cochrane and others) and here we are now talking about how it needs to change. It also feels as if evidence-based medicine still has to convince a large section of the wider public (along with some healthcare professionals) of its advantages. The maturity of an approach, paradigm or philosophy can be measured in how it adapts to changing priorities and needs. Evidence-based medicine is surely now at or approaching that maturity.

Outside of the practice of evidence-based medicine itself there are other movements that will affect how medicine is practised in the coming decades. There are several movements within science and society that will affect the future of evidence-based medicine. There is a growing unease with the medicalisation of normal variations. Try answering the question of 'what is normal?' – there are always people who fall outside any widely accepted definition and who do not have a medical condition. An obvious example of this is in blood tests: the normal range often covers two or three standard deviations but this still leaves some people who will naturally be outside the normal range without having a medical problem.

There is an argument that many 'diseases' are part of the normal ageing process and are not a medical problem in themselves. An example would be chronic kidney disease. There is a debate over whether we are not diagnosing enough or whether we are overdiagnosing people with CKD. The vast majority of people diagnosed with CKD will have no significant impact on their quality of life if left untreated. By treating a large cohort of people with medication for CKD, we are medicalising them and potentially decreasing their quality of life unnecessarily.

A debate is also taking place over whether screening programmes overdiagnose. We are all taught the United Nations criteria for screening programmes, known as the Wilson and Jungner criteria (*see* Chapter 6). These criteria exist to try to ensure that screening programmes are effectively evaluated and produce more good than harm. However, there is growing evidence that some screening programmes are more harmful than helpful. The breast cancer screening programme has been subject to much debate. The overtreatment of some women with ductal carcinoma in situ that would never have had an impact on their health and may even have resolved without any intervention is a real concern – it is certainly reducing the quality of life of some women. The counterargument is based on how much harm is acceptable if lives are saved.

Another development that has been slowly making ground over recent years is personalised medicine based on DNA analysis. If it is known that people with certain DNA traits or mutations are more likely to develop a particular disease, then treatment can be targeted at either early detection or even prevention. If a DNA-based trait means that a particular group of people will not have any benefit from a certain medication, then you would not knowingly give that group that medication. There are a great many hopes that better understanding of DNA mutations may help treat and prevent disease. It is possible that this will become much more important in our day-to-day practice within a few decades, particularly when linked to another development: big data.

Big data refers to the vast and growing databases that gather all sorts of information about individuals and groups. Recent advances in information technology, computing and data analysis mean that these vast quantities of data can be used to provide very detailed knowledge of specific phenomena. Imagine knowing in great detail how disease prevalence varies across a country and how that could result in targeting resources into preventive measures or into better treatment in those areas that need it. Imagine having enough data to see how individual choices affect health outcomes. The possibility for incredibly detailed and useful epidemiological studies is immense.

Having large data sets that show how patients react to certain drugs can help us understand, in conjunction with data sets of DNA, who would benefit most from receiving particular drugs and who should not receive that drug. The possibilities of big data are vast and will almost certainly change medicine and push it in new directions. Even the basic medical art of history, examination and investigation may be irreversibly altered by algorithms and systems that help with diagnosis based on data input and computing power. It could be that tests will be chosen based on how useful they are calculated to be – if there is uncertainty then the diagnostic power of a test (based on calculated likelihood ratios) can be determined and only the most useful tests ordered.

However, the 'elephant in the room' is the cost of all these innovations. Healthcare is incredibly expensive and many countries are struggling with paying for it, alongside rising expectations and increased access to healthcare provision. Evidence is needed that these innovations are cost-effective and it is possible that organisations such as the National Health Service in the UK will not be able to afford to finance many innovations.

Drug companies are a vital part of healthcare but there has been, on occasions, a strained relationship with public sector organisations such as the National Health Service. The marketing of drugs can alter the perceptions of healthcare professionals and lead to non-evidence-based prescribing. There is a need for full disclosure of all trial results. The Cochrane review on the antiviral drugs Relenza and Tamiflu found that when all the data were looked at, the evidence for using these drugs was significantly watered down.* Drug companies have large research and development budgets and may be able to pay for some innovations but will be more likely to target those with the largest potential returns. There have been suggestions of centrally organised research budgets, with governments and drug companies working together to set priorities and allocate funding to research.

Given the discussion outlined here, it should be clear that we all need to understand and incorporate evidence-based medicine into our daily practice in

---

* Torjesen I. Cochrane review questions effectiveness of neuraminidase inhibitors. *BMJ.* 2014; **348**: g2675.

order to be able to discern how it may best help our practice. This is also necessary in order for us to keep abreast of challenges and changes within medicine. Ultimately, any system to improve medical outcomes for our patients has to be welcomed as well as challenged so that its limits are found.

Dr David Sackett and colleagues, in their seminal editorial in the *BMJ* from 1996, summed up both what evidence-based medicine is and how it cannot be the only skill a clinician needs. Evidence-based medicine is the 'conscientious, explicit and judicious use of current best evidence in making decisions about the care of individual patients'. They go on to say that 'without clinical expertise, practice risks becoming tyrannised by evidence, for even excellent external evidence may be inapplicable to or inappropriate for an individual patient'.*

---

* Sackett DL, Rosenberg WM, Gray JA, *et al*. Evidence based medicine: what it is and what it isn't. *BMJ*. 1996; **312**(7023): 71–2.

CHAPTER 9

Practice questions

Q 9.1 Which of the following statements are *true* regarding descriptive statistics?
a) They are used to summarise the characteristics of study participants.
b) They give results from a sample group that are generalisable to the whole population.
c) They include such methods as the chi-squared test, regression and analysis of variance.
d) They include methods such as averages, measures of spread and deviation.
e) They are particularly useful if you wish to apply the results of your study to a larger population.

Q 9.2 Ethnographic research aims to:
a) understand the things that people write
b) get people's views through interviews
c) solve a problem through the use of research
d) develop an understanding of a particular group of people through the researcher immersing themselves in the activities of the group
e) explore phenomena through the experiences and perceptions of individuals through interviews, observation and discussion.

Q 9.3 Work out the disability-adjusted life year (DALY) if a patient is diagnosed with a terminal disease at the age of 70 and his life expectancy before diagnosis would have been 80 years. He dies aged 76 but he has greatly reduced quality of life for the last 2 years of his life. This reduced quality of life is quantified as being half of a normal quality of life. He also experienced slightly reduced quality of life between diagnosis and onset of deterioration at the age of 74. This was quantified as a reduction in quality of life of 5%. Write your answer in the box provided.

Q 9.4 Focus groups can give useful data and information, but which of the following is a limitation of focus groups?
a) They are moderated so the discussion can be kept on track.
b) They produce a limited amount of data.
c) They are simple to conduct and finding participants is easy.
d) Participants in a group tend to agree and state socially acceptable views.
e) The data produced is easily generalisable.

Q 9.5 Choose the *single most appropriate* answer. Qualitative interviewing is:
a) structured with responses having to be on a measurable scale
b) open to changes in the discussion topic
c) a wide variety of techniques that aim to uncover people's experiences and values
d) carefully controlled so that participants cannot change the topic

Q 9.6 A research study is looking to reach a conclusion regarding exposure to environmental pollution and the risk of asthma in children. It will combine the results from many previous studies. Which is the *single most appropriate* study design? Select *one* option only.
a) Case-control study
b) Cohort study
c) Correlation study
d) Qualitative study
e) Meta-analysis

Q 9.7 A research study is proposed to look at likely causative factors for a rare disease with a suspected long lag time between exposure and developing the disease. Which of the following is the *most appropriate* study design?
a) Case-control study
b) Cohort study
c) Randomised controlled trial
d) Qualitative study
e) Meta-analysis

Q 9.8 What would be the *most appropriate* outcome measure for the study in Question 9.7?
a) quality-adjusted life year (QALY)
b) Treatment effect
c) Odds ratio
d) Forest plot
e) Categorical data or description
f) Relative risk increase

Q 9.9 A hazard ratio of one implies what?
a) The difference between two groups is significant
b) That one treatment is twice as harmful as the other
c) That one treatment is less harmful than the other
d) That both treatments are harmful
e) That there is no difference in risk between the two treatments

Q 9.10 Which of the following statements are *true* regarding inferential statistics?
a) They are used to summarise the characteristics of study participants.
b) They give results from a sample group that are generalisable to the whole population.
c) They include such methods as the chi-squared test, regression and analysis of variance.
d) They include methods such as averages, measures of spread and deviation.
e) They are useful if you wish to apply the results of your study to a larger population.

Q 9.11 Which of the following is the *most appropriate outcome* for a meta-analysis?
a) quality-adjusted life year (QALY)
b) Hazard ratio
c) Odds ratio
d) Forest plot
e) Relative risk

Q 9.12 What are funnel plots primarily used for?
a) To demonstrate the power of a meta-analysis
b) To demonstrate the existence of publication bias in meta-analyses
c) To provide a graphical representation of the relative risk results in a case-control study
d) To provide a graphical representation of the relative risk results in a cohort study
e) To provide a graphical representation of the probability of a patient experiencing an adverse effect

Q 9.13 What does 'grounded theory' refer to?
a) Theoretical ideas and concepts emerge from the data as they are collected.
b) Theories should be tested with controlled trials.
c) Theoretical ideas and concepts should be applied to the data once they have all been collected.
d) Theory should be easy to understand.
e) Theory that ensures that any found relationships are explained clearly and simply.

Q 9.14 If a study quotes a 95% confidence interval, which *one* of the following statements is *true*?
a) There is a 95% chance of the true value for the population lying outside these limits.
b) There is a 5% chance of the true value for the population lying outside these limits.
c) There is a 2.5% chance of the true value for the population lying outside these limits.
d) There is a minus 5% chance of the true value for the population lying outside these limits.
e) There is a 5% chance that the study is flawed in its design.

Q 9.15 Match the following terms (left) with the *most appropriate* definition (right).

a) Sensitivity

1) The likelihood that a given test result would be expected in a patient with the target disorder compared with the likelihood that that same result would be expected in a patient without the target disorder

b) Specificity

2) The proportion of patients with the disorder of interest who have a positive test result

c) Positive predictive value

3) The proportion of patients without the disorder of interest who have a negative test result

d) Negative predictive value

4) Proportion of those with positive test results who have the disease of interest

e) Likelihood ratio

5) Proportion of those with negative test results who do not have the disease of interest

Q 9.16 Which *one* of the following formulas is used to calculate the likelihood ratio for a positive test result?

a) $\dfrac{\text{sensitivity}}{1 - \text{specificity}}$

b) $\dfrac{1 - \text{sensitivity}}{\text{specificity}}$

c) $\dfrac{\text{TN}}{(\text{TN} + \text{FN})}$

d) $\dfrac{\text{TN}}{(\text{TN} + \text{FP})}$

e) $\dfrac{\text{TP}}{(\text{TP} + \text{FN})}$

f) $\dfrac{\text{TP}}{(\text{TP} + \text{FP})}$

Q **9.17** You are reading a research paper regarding a new blood test that can be used to screen for a cancer. The new blood test was compared with a gold standard test. It was found that out of 4400 people studied, 1760 people with the disease were correctly identified and 1320 people without the disease were correctly identified as not having the disease. However, 880 people with a positive test did not have the disease. What is the *specificity* of this new test as a percentage?

a) 20%
b) 33%
c) 60%
d) 66%
e) 75%
f) 80%

Q **9.18** What is the *sensitivity* of this test as a percentage?
a) 20%
b) 33%
c) 60%
d) 66%
e) 75%
f) 80%

Q **9.19** What is the *positive predictive value* as a percentage?
a) 20%
b) 33%
c) 60%
d) 66%
e) 75%
f) 80%

Q **9.20** What is the *negative predictive value* as a percentage?
a) 20%
b) 33%
c) 60%
d) 66%
e) 75%
f) 80%

Q 9.21 What is the *likelihood ratio for a positive test result?*
a) 0.1
b) 0.2
c) 0.3
d) 1
e) 2

Q 9.22 What is the *likelihood ratio for a negative test result?*
a) 0.1
b) 0.2
c) 0.3
d) 1
e) 2

Q 9.23 A cohort study is conducted to evaluate the relationship between statin use and pancreatic cancer. The study examines the pancreatic cancer rate in 3500 people taking statins and 4000 people not taking statins over 5 years. Over the 5-year period, 35 people taking statins and 42 people not taking statins develop pancreatic cancer. What is the *risk* of pancreatic cancer in the group taking statins?
a) 0.01
b) 0.05
c) 0.1
d) 0.5
e) 1.0

Q 9.24 What is the *risk ratio?* Select *one* option only.
a) 0.01
b) 0.95
c) 0.1
d) 0.90
e) 1.0

Q 9.25 A randomised controlled trial looking at the management of hypertension divides its subjects into two groups: Group A, with 15 836 subjects, receives a new antihypertensive medication; Group B, with 16 164 subjects, receives standard treatment. After 2 years the risk of a stroke is 14.6% for those taking the new medication, while for those on standard treatment it is 5.6%. The trial is stopped and the new drug withdrawn from the market. Calculate the number needed to harm (NNH) for the new medication to cause one extra stroke.

a) 0.1
b) 10
c) 11
d) 110
e) 2

a) Descriptive statistics
b) Inferential statistics
c) Statistical significance
d) The null hypothesis
e) P-value

For each definition given in Questions 9.26–9.30, select the *single most likely* option from the list above.

Q 9.26 That a result is unlikely to have arisen by chance

Q 9.27 Summarise data and enable quicker understanding of what the data represent

Q 9.28 The chance of obtaining a result, at least as extreme, if the null hypothesis were true

Q 9.29 The hypothesis that there is no relationship between variables

Q 9.30 Are used to make conclusions based on the available data but those conclusions reach beyond what the data themselves show

Q 9.31 Results are deemed to be significant if the p-value is?
a) <0.01
b) >0.01
c) <0.02
d) >0.05
e) <0.05

Q 9.32 A research study looking at a new antihypertensive, drug A, has the null hypothesis that there is no difference in blood pressure reduction between drug A and standard treatment, drug B. The research project does not have adequate power and reports that there was no difference. It is later discovered that there is a difference in blood pressure reduction between these two drugs. What error has the research study displayed?
a) Type I
b) Type II
c) Both type I and type II
d) Neither type I nor type II
e) A type of bias

Q 9.33 The power of a research project is the probability that it would detect a statistically significant difference between two variables. Which option also represents the power of a study?
a) 1– probability of a type I error
b) 1+ probability of a type II error
c) 1– probability of a type II error
d) 1+ probability of a type II error
e) None of the above

a) Validity

b) Reliability

c) Accuracy

d) Probability

e) Generalisability

For each definition given in Questions 9.34–9.39, which is the *single most likely option* from the list above?

Q 9.34 How likely the results from a study are to be replicated in similar, repeated studies

Q 9.35 The degree to which the study results are appropriately inferred and measure what they are intended to measure

Q 9.36 Whether the results of a study can be applied beyond the study sample and context

Q 9.37 The measure of how likely an event is to occur

Q 9.38 How close we are to measuring what we aimed to measure

Q 9.39 Which *one* of the following answers is *not* true? The median is:

a) the value that falls in the middle of a data set if all the values are put in order of size

b) often used to describe skewed distributions

c) the same as the mean and mode in a normal distribution

d) usually greater than the mean in a negatively skewed distribution

e) usually less than the mode in a positively skewed distribution

a) Scatter diagram
b) Box plot
c) Forest plot
d) Funnel plot
e) Histogram

For each definition given in Questions 9.40–9.44, which is the single most likely option from the above list?

Q 9.40   This shows continuous data such as interval or ratio data. It also shows the distribution of data within ranges.

Q 9.41   A common way of representing the results of a meta-analysis. It shows the size or weighting of the study, the confidence interval for the results of each trial and an overall result combining the results of all the selected trials.

Q 9.42   This can plot data that have two variables for each measurement; maintaining the relationship between the two by using the x-axis and y-axis.

Q 9.43   This shows the distribution of interval data, with its central value and variability also shown. It is useful for comparing two or more data sets.

Q 9.44   This is a graph that is particularly useful in systematic reviews and meta-analysis to look for evidence that not all data have been published.

Q 9.45 Choose *one* answer from the following options. The standard error of the mean is?

a) A measure of the variation between values
b) The difference between the mean and the median
c) The difference between the mean and the mode
d) The difference between the means of two data sets
e) A measure of the accuracy of the sample mean to the true population mean

Q 9.46 Which *one* answer is *not correct* when considering confidence intervals?

a) If a confidence interval of 95% is used, then the true population parameter is 95% likely to fall within that range.
b) If the confidence interval crosses the line of no effect (ARR or RRR = 0% or RR or OR =1), then the study has not found a significant difference between parameters.
c) If the confidence interval is narrow, then the study probably has reasonable power to detect an effect.
d) The 95% confidence interval limits can be calculated using mean $\pm$ (1.96 $\times$ SEM), where SEM is the standard error of the mean.
e) One in 25 significant findings will be spurious.

Q 9.47 A GP wishes to assess if there is a correlation between her patients' blood pressure and their fasting blood glucose. Assuming both are distributed normally, which statistical test could be used?

a) Chi-squared test
b) Mann–Whitney U test
c) Student's t-test
d) Spearman's rank correlation coefficient
e) Pearson's product-moment correlation coefficient

Q 9.48 Which test is *not* used in non-normally distributed (non-parametric) data?

a) Mann–Whitney U test
b) Student's t-test
c) Spearman's rank correlation coefficient
d) Linear regression
e) Chi-squared test

Q **9.49** The Department of Health wishes to see if mammographic screening results in increased survival from breast cancer. Assuming that
the study is well performed, what is the *most likely* form of bias?

a) Lead-time bias
b) Selection bias
c) Spectrum bias
d) Recall bias
e) Procedure bias

a) Simple random sampling
b) Stratified sampling
c) Quota sampling
d) Cluster sampling
e) Opportunity sampling

For each of the numbered gaps in Questions 9.50 and 9.51, select *one* option
from the list above to complete the definitions.

Q **9.50** If the population is large it sometimes helps to split it into groups
and then sample from those smaller groups. This splitting can happen several times and is called _____.

Q **9.51** _____ is undertaken by splitting the population into subgroups
with similar characteristics and then taking a sample that includes
members from all subgroups.

a) Grounded theory
b) Phenomenology
c) Ethnography
d) Action research
e) Pragmatic research

For each definition given in Questions 9.52–9.56, select the single most likely option from the list above.

Q 9.52 Tries to avoid preconceived ideas and instead allows theories to develop from research data

Q 9.53 Does not use a single, neat qualitative research methodology but uses several methods to gain in-depth understanding

Q 9.54 Aims to solve a problem while the research is in progress

Q 9.55 This is a systematic study of a social group or culture using a number of methods undertaken as fieldwork

Q 9.56 This is the study of subjective experience to help understand how people think about something

Q 9.57 Which method is *not* considered to be a qualitative research method?
a) Participant observation
b) Narrative-based research
c) Socratic method
d) Focus groups
e) Delphi technique

Q 9.58–9.62 Match the appropriate study type to the number in the hierarchy of evidence.

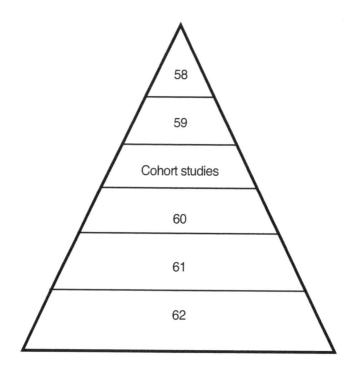

a) Expert opinion
b) Case-control study
c) Systematic reviews and meta-analyses
d) Case series and case studies
e) Randomised controlled trials

Q 9.63 A university department of general practice wishes to assess the mental health effects of taking 'legal highs' over time. What would be the *most suitable* type of research study?

a) Randomised controlled trial
b) Case-control study
c) Systematic review
d) Cohort study
e) Cross-sectional survey

Q 9.64 A study, looking at a population of 18- to 25-year-olds who have used cannabis regularly over 10 years found that in the population of 200 cannabis users, 20 developed symptoms of anxiety. Out of the control group of 200 people, two developed anxiety. What is the absolute risk reduction?

a) 0.09
b) 0.1
c) 0.01
d) 10
e) 18

Q 9.65 A new drug to prevent gout is developed. In a study to assess its effect, 1000 people were given the new drug and 20 developed gout. In the control group of 800 who took a placebo, 40 developed gout. What is the relative risk reduction?

a) 0.05
b) 0.03
c) 0.02
d) 0.4
e) 0.6

Q 9.66 What is the calculation for the number needed to treat (where CER is the control event rate and EER is the experimental event rate)?

a) CER/EER
b) 1/CER – EER
c) CER – EER/CER
d) 1/CER
e) 1/EER

Q 9.67 In a randomised controlled trial comparing aspirin with a new drug in patients with ischaemic heart disease, 1000 people receive the new drug, of whom 20 experience significant side effects; in the group of 800 receiving aspirin, four experience significant side effects. What is the number needed to harm (NNH) when using the new drug as compared with aspirin?

a) 66.6
b) 33.3
c) 0.015
d) 0.02
e) 50

Q 9.68 A cohort study compares the development of deep vein thromboses (DVTs) in patients taking the combined oral contraceptive (COC) pill. Of the 800 women taking the COC, four develop a DVT. In the control group of 1000 women not taking the COC pill, there is one DVT. What is the relative risk for a woman who takes the COC pill?

a) 5
b) 0.005
c) 0.001
d) 0.004
e) 2

Q 9.69 A case-control study looking at radon gas exposure of over $100\,Bqm^{-3}$ in people with lung cancer found the following result. What is the odds ratio of people exposed to radon gas developing lung cancer?

	Lung cancer present	No lung cancer	Total population
Exposure to radon	10	9990	10000
No exposure	2	9998	10000

a) 2
b) 3
c) 5
d) 10
e) 20

Q **9.70** An odds ratio is the usual outcome from which type of study?
a) Systematic review
b) Cohort study
c) Case-control study
d) Case series
e) Cross-sectional survey

Q **9.71** A study to look at the risk of asbestos exposure in people who smoked, over a 20-year period, yielded the following results. What is the odds ratio of people who smoke and are exposed to asbestos developing lung cancer?

	Lung cancer present	Lung cancer not present	Population
Exposure to asbestos	130	870	1000
No exposure to asbestos	80	720	800

a) 1.63
b) 1.21
c) 0.8
d) 0.15
e) 1.34

Q **9.72** Which one of the following points is *not* an advantage of undertaking a cohort study?
a) Often cheaper and easier than a randomised controlled trial
b) Can study causal relationships
c) Normally randomised or blinded
d) Can determine risk factors for disease
e) Multiple outcomes can be studied

Q **9.73** Which one of the following is *not* an advantage of a case-control study?
a) Cheaper and easier to conduct than randomised controlled trials and cohort studies
b) Look prospectively
c) Can be conducted by small teams
d) Can be used for rare diseases
e) Usually a preliminary study to consider associations

Use the following contingency table to answer Questions 9.74–9.76.

	Condition present	Condition absent
Test positive	TP	FP
Test negative	FN	TN

Q 9.74 Which of the following formulas is used to calculate the specificity of a screening test?
a) TN/TN + FP
b) TN/FP
c) TN/TN + FN
d) TP/FP + TN
e) TP/FN + TN

Q 9.75 Which of the following formulas is used to calculate the positive predictive value?
a) TP/TP + FP
b) FP/TP + FP
c) TP/TP + FN
d) TP/FP + TN
e) TP/FP

Q 9.76 Which of the following formulas is used to calculate the sensitivity?
a) FP/TN + FP
b) FN/TN + FP
c) TP/TP + FP
d) TP/TP + FN
e) TN/TN + FP

Q 9.77 A new blood test is created to diagnose a pulmonary embolism. Two hundred patients presenting with pleuritic chest pain to an accident and emergency department have a computed tomography pulmonary angiogram performed. Forty are confirmed to have a pulmonary embolism. The new test was positive in 30 of the confirmed cases. The new test was also positive in 20 of the remaining 160. What is the positive predictive value?
a) 0.75
b) 60%
c) 15%
d) 93.3%
e) 0.875

Q 9.78 What is the formula for calculating the likelihood ratio for a negative result?

a) Sensitivity/1 – specificity
b) Sensitivity/specificity
c) Specificity/sensitivity
d) 1 – sensitivity/specificity
e) 1 – specificity/sensitivity

Q 9.79 A genetic screening test is developed to assess the risk of developing hypertension. In a population of 1000 people, 250 developed hypertension. The genetic screening test detected 200 of these. Of the remaining 750, the test was positive in 100 people. What was the sensitivity of the genetic screening test?

a) 86.67%
b) 66.67%
c) 20%
d) 72%
e) 80%

Q 9.80 Which answer is *not* one of the 10 Wilson and Jungner screening principles?

a) The condition should be an important health problem.
b) There should be an accepted treatment for patients with the disease.
c) There should be a known mortality rate associated with the condition.
d) There should be a recognisable latent or early symptomatic stage.
e) The cost of case finding should be economically balanced in relation to possible expenditure on medical care as a whole.

Q 9.81 What is the definition of infant mortality?

a) The annual number of deaths among babies less than 28 days old
b) The number of deaths in a specified population in a specified time
c) The annual number of deaths among children 1–4 years old
d) The percentage of people alive at a specified time after diagnosis
e) The annual number of deaths among children under 1 year of age

Q 9.82 Which *one* acronym represents a method of formulating a question about the clinical care of a patient?
a) DALY
b) PICO
c) NICE
d) QALY
e) NIHR

Q 9.83 Which *one* statement is *not* true for QALYs?
a) Stands for quality-adjusted life years
b) Cannot be used to determine cost-effectiveness
c) One QALY is a year of life gained with 'perfect' health
d) Takes into account the expected life expectancy of a person
e) Takes into account the number of additional years of life expected from a treatment

Q 9.84 What is post-test probability a measure of?
a) It is similar to the incidence of a disease
b) It is similar to the prevalence of a disease
c) The likelihood of an individual testing positive or negative for a disease
d) The risk to an individual of contracting a disease
e) The probability of a patient dying from the disease in a specified time

ANSWERS TO QUESTIONS IN CHAPTER 9

Note that questions in other chapters have full answers and explanations within the text of the chapter.

A 9.1	a, d		A 9.43	b
A 9.2	d		A 9.44	d
A 9.3	5.2 years		A 9.45	e
A 9.4	d		A 9.46	e
A 9.5	c		A 9.47	e
A 9.6	e		A 9.48	b
A 9.7	a		A 9.49	a
A 9.8	c		A 9.50	d
A 9.9	e		A 9.51	b
A 9.10	b, c, e		A 9.52	a
A 9.11	d		A 9.53	e
A 9.12	b		A 9.54	d
A 9.13	a		A 9.55	c
A 9.14	b		A 9.56	b
A 9.15	1e, 2a, 3b, 4c, 5d		A 9.57	c
A 9.16	a		A 9.58	c
A 9.17	c		A 9.59	e
A 9.18	f		A 9.60	b
A 9.19	d		A 9.61	d
A 9.20	e		A 9.62	a
A 9.21	e		A 9.63	d
A 9.22	c		A 9.64	a
A 9.23	a		A 9.65	e
A 9.24	b		A 9.66	b
A 9.25	c		A 9.67	a
A 9.26	c		A 9.68	a
A 9.27	a		A 9.69	c
A 9.28	e		A 9.70	c
A 9.29	d		A 9.71	e
A 9.30	b		A 9.72	c
A 9.31	e		A 9.73	b
A 9.32	b		A 9.74	a
A 9.33	c		A 9.75	a
A 9.34	b		A 9.76	d

A 9.35	a		A 9.77	b
A 9.36	e		A 9.78	d
A 9.37	d		A 9.79	e
A 9.38	c		A 9.80	c
A 9.39	e		A 9.81	e
A 9.40	e		A 9.82	b
A 9.41	c		A 9.83	b
A 9.42	a		A 9.84	c

Glossary

absolute risk   The probability that an individual will experience the outcome of interest during a specified period of time.

absolute risk reduction   The difference in risk between two groups.

accuracy   How close a statistic (sample value) is to the true (population) value it is attempting to measure.

association   Similar to correlation, one variable is related to another – as one changes so does the other.

Bayesian   An approach to statistics that assigns probability to events or parameters before data collection and refines these after data collection. This approach allows reasoning about events that are not known to have occurred yet, and it can allow for subjective beliefs to be incorporated into a model.

bias   Errors in a study design that affect the final result, meaning the study does not accurately measure what it set out to measure.

blinding   Methods to ensure the participants and researchers are unaware of who receives which study intervention.

case-control   A study that compares people with an outcome of interest and people who do not have that outcome.

categorical data   Data that can be sorted into categories.

cohort study   A longitudinal observational study where a group of people are followed over time.

confidence interval   An estimated range of values within which an unknown population parameter is likely to be.

confounding variable   A variable that correlates with both the variables being studied but which has not been accounted for in the research design.

contingency table   A table summarising relationships between categories.

continuous data   Data that can be counted, ordered and measured because the data can fall on any value within an interval.

control group   The comparison group, which is not subject to intervention.

correlation   A measure of the relationship between two or more variables.

correlation coefficient A measure of how closely related two variables are, it takes a value between −1 and +1.

crossover study Study participants are subject to two treatments one after the other.

cross-sectional study Study done at a single point in time across a population of interest.

DALY Disability-adjusted life year; life years and quality of life *lost* to disability. One DALY equals 1 year of healthy life lost.

Delphi technique A structured forecasting method utilising a panel of experts.

dependent variable The variable that changes as the independent variable is manipulated.

effectiveness A measure of the benefit resulting from an intervention under usual conditions of clinical care.

efficacy A measure of the benefit resulting from an intervention under ideal conditions.

ethnography A detailed description of a group of people based on detailed observation of those people.

event rate The rate of occurrence of an outcome that is being studied.

focus group A group of people brought together to discuss a specified topic with a moderator present.

generalisability Whether the results of a study can be applied beyond the study sample or context.

grounded theory Theory that arises from the research findings.

hazard The rate at which events happen. Often related to survival analysis, so the hazard may be death or morbidity over a defined period of time.

hazard ratio The risk of an event over time in one group compared with the risk of an event over time in a comparison group. Also known as the relative hazard.

heterogeneity Systematic differences between the results of studies in a meta-analysis due to methodological and sampling differences.

homogeneity A measure of the similarity between studies based on the characteristics of study participants and the methods used.

incidence The number of new cases of a condition occurring over a specified time frame in a specified population.

inclusion/exclusion criteria Attributes that are either sought or avoided in research participants – particularly in qualitative research but also within drug trials, for example.

independent events Two or more events that have no influence on each other.

independent variable   The variable that is manipulated to cause an effect in the dependent variable.

inductive reasoning   Drawing conclusions that apply more widely from a limited sample or data set.

likelihood   A measure of the extent to which a sample provides support for particular values of a parameter.

likelihood ratio   The likelihood that a given test result would be expected in a patient with the target disorder compared with the likelihood that that same result would be expected in a patient without the target disorder.

mean   The arithmetical average of the observed values.

median   The middle value if the observed values are placed in order.

meta-analysis   Statistical techniques for summarising the results of several studies.

mode   The value that occurs most frequently in a data set.

negative predictive value   Proportion of those with negative test results who do not have the disease of interest.

nominal data   Data that cannot have a meaningful number attached.

non-parametric distribution   A data set that is not normally distributed.

normal distribution   A symmetrical distribution around the mean with a bell shape when plotted.

null hypothesis   The hypothesis that there is no association between variables.

number needed to harm   The number of patients who need to be treated before one additional adverse outcome occurs due to the treatment.

number needed to treat   The number of patients who need to be treated to prevent one additional bad outcome. Also known as the number needed to treat to benefit one (NNTB).

odds   The proportion of events to non-events – for example, 2:1.

odds ratio   The odds of an event happening in the treatment group compared with the odds of the event happening in the control group.

ordinal data   Data with a meaningful order but in which the distance between points is not the same.

outlier   An extreme value that differs greatly from the other data values.

parameter   The true value for a population – this is estimated by statistics from studies.

pilot study   An initial small-scale study used to evaluate the practicalities of performing a larger study and to check that the methods used are suitable. Also used to estimate an appropriate sample size before starting a larger study.

placebo   A neutral intervention, often administered to a control group.

population   Every member of the group that a research study is looking at.

positive predictive value   Proportion of those with positive test results who have the disease of interest.

power   The ability of a test to reject the null hypothesis when it is actually false.

precision   How likely a result is to be replicated by other studies under the same conditions.

prevalence   The proportion of people with a disease at a given time in a specified population.

probability   A quantitative measure of how likely an event is to occur, given pre-existing knowledge of the conditions that give rise to the event.

p-value   The probability of obtaining a result by chance at least as extreme as the one observed, assuming there is no relationship between the variables studied.

QALY   Quality-adjusted life year; a measure of health *improvement* in terms of years of life *gained*, adjusted for quality of life. One QALY equals 1 year of perfect health gained.

quantile   A set of points that divide a data set into groups of equal size – for example, a quartile cuts the group into four equal groups.

randomised controlled trial   An experimental study that randomly allocates participants to intervention or control.

range   The difference between the largest and the smallest observed values.

relative risk   The ratio of risk in one group to risk in another group – one divided by the other.

relative risk reduction   The proportional reduction in rates of adverse events between experimental and control groups.

reliability   How likely the results from a study are to be replicated in similar, repeated studies.

risk ratio   This is the same as relative risk – the risk of an event in one group divided by the risk of the event in another group.

risk reduction   Either absolute or relative changes in risk.

sample   A group drawn from the population of interest.

sampling   Techniques for recruiting participants to a study when it is not practicable to involve the complete population.

sensitivity   The proportion of patients with the disorder of interest who have a positive test result.

significance level   The probability of wrongly rejecting the null hypothesis, commonly set at 0.05.

skew   Asymmetry in the distribution of data values.

specificity   The proportion of patients without the disorder of interest who have a negative test result.

standard deviation A measure of the spread of data either side of the mean or median.

standard error An estimate of the standard deviation of a statistic (value found from a sample) if a study were to be repeated.

standardised mortality rate Mortality rates adjusted for the composition of the populations being compared.

statistic A value that is calculated from a sample, it is an estimate of the population parameter.

statistics Inductive reasoning to discover the nature of the world based on observations.

systematic review A review in which all the relevant trials on a topic are summarised according to predetermined criteria.

trends Changes in variables of interest over time.

triangulation Using two or more methods in a study to ensure the results are as accurate as possible.

type I error Wrongly rejecting the null hypothesis.

type II error Wrongly accepting the null hypothesis.

validity The degree to which the study results are appropriately inferred and measure what they intended to measure.

Index

absolute risk (AR) 74–8, 155
accuracy
  and precision 22
  and significance 19
Acheson Report 91
action research 54–5
age-standardised mortality rates 113
AKT (Applied Knowledge Test)
  marking of 8
  pass rates for 8–9
  preparation for 3–5, 11–12
  question formats 6–7
  revising for 9–11
  succeeding in 133
algorithms 7, 11, 80, 138
AllTrials 129
ambiguity, avoiding 57
Applied Knowledge Test Content Guide 4,
  10, 12, 90
attrition 80
audit cycle 121–2
averages 17
axes (x and y) 31, 33–6, 67, 69

bar charts 24, 31, 33–5
baseline figures 75
Bayes' theorem 107
Bayesian methods 132
bias
  in case reports 87
  examining evidence for 123
  inevitability of 54
  in meta-analyses 68
  in RCT 72
  sources of 48, 51
  in systematic reviews 66
  types of 43–4, 152

big data 138
bimodal distributions 28
bivariate data 36
Black Report 91
blinding, in RCTs 73; *see also*
  double-blinding
BMJ Evidence Centre 126
box plots 31, 35–6
British National Formulary 10

case-control studies 80–3, 107, 156–7
case reports 64, 86–7
case series 86–7
categorical data 31, 33–5
Cates plot 130–1
causality, establishing 39, 80, 83
cause-specific survival 113
censuses 17
central tendency, measures of 27–8
CER (control event rate) 74–5, 77–8,
  80–1, 155
chi-squared test 42
child mortality rate 112, 114
Clark, Sally 14–15
Clinical Knowledge Summaries 124
Clinical Practice Research Datalink 126–7
Clinical Skills Assessment 5–6
clinical trials; *see also* RCTs
  application to practice 135–6
  publication of results 129
closed questions 57
cluster sampling 49–50
Cochrane, Archie 1, 125, 136
Cochrane reviews 9, 64, 125, 134, 138
cohort studies 79–81
  and hierarchy of evidence 64
  practice questions on 146, 156–7

CPD with Radcliffe

You can now use a selection of our books to achieve CPD (Continuing Professional Development) points through directed reading.

We provide a free online form and downloadable certificate for your appraisal portfolio. Look for the CPD logo and register with us at: www.radcliffehealth.com/cpd

CERTIFIED
The CPD Certification
Service